A Message from
Kelly and Claire

Let's start at the beginning, where it all began. We are two ordinary people, with extraordinary gifts. We have always had a natural ability to connect to energies in the room and we grew up in ordinary homes, went to ordinary schools and had, you've guessed it, ordinary jobs.

But we all reach a pivotal point in our lives where something shakes you, and we knew after losing people very dear to us, that life was for living, not just going from a to b and doing what is necessary in the day - school runs, grocery shopping and work.

We have always had a passion for astrology, lunar energies and all things magical. We also had a dream of having daughters. From an early age we were always very maternal, we daydreamed of bows, pink glitter and unicorn sparkles. And you don't think "what if it never happens?" It doesn't cross your mind; you plan in your mind how your future family will look and that is your life mapped out for you.

But this isn't the reality. You don't just get what you daydream of, which we were going to find out when we did become mothers, with five boys between us. They are absolutely everything and more. But a dream can be anything personal to you, and this was ours.

We are both naturally passionate people, our signs being a mix of Aquarius and Aries. When it comes to astrological compatibility, Aquarius and Aries have a strong connection right out the gate. Aquarius is an air sign that brings intelligence, depth and originality to relationships. Aries is a fire sign teeming with passion, persistence and excitement in creating something original. Both signs are hardworking and don't give up!

Together, we aren't daunted by challenges. This makes the perfect combination of creative, determined, intuitive personalities with a sprinkling of stubbornness. So, we weren't about to let that daydream slip by without giving it our best shot. And that's what we did.

We met in 2021, and from there we discussed everything we had learnt within the natural gender selection world over the last 14 years. We immediately had the same train of thought, and we set about making the best possible method to bring that manifestation into a reality. We enrolled in astrology courses, invested hundreds of pounds in research and we stayed up all night for months on end. We looked at absolutely everything and we cross-checked it, studied it and looked for patterns.

Our astrological research spanned 4 years (I told you we were stubborn) and it became more than a hobby, it was our passion, our love and we really came into ourselves, with an "Ahaaaa" lightbulb moment. This is where we were always supposed to be, this is our calling, our destiny and everything we are as people. We are cosmic, it is our higher self, our extra child, it is all of our attributes, skills and natural abilities rolled into one.

And so, in November 2021, we made our Facebook page and set about sharing with the world the amazing method that had stolen our hearts. With us being open to spirituality and working within the field of fertility daily alongside astrology and astronomy, we can guide you on all aspects of our method via this book. We want to share with you our method so you too can harness these lunar energies and use the Moon's magick to fulfil your dreams, like we did.

Let us take you by the hand, and let the Moon, and us, be your guide.

x x

KELLY LOUISE HILL
AND
CLAIRE LILLEY-WINDUST

THE COSMIC SWAY METHOD

CHOOSE THE SEX OF YOUR NEXT BABY

A NATURAL GENDER SELECTION GUIDE,
BACKED BY SCIENTIFIC RESEARCH
AND OUR EXCLUSIVE TIMING METHODOLOGY

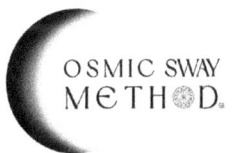

First published in paperback by
Michael Terence Publishing in 2024
www.mtp.agency

Copyright © 2024
Cosmic Sway Method LTD
www.cosmicswaymethod.com

Kelly Louise Hill and Claire Lilley-Windust
have asserted the right to be identified as
the authors of this work in accordance with the
Copyright, Designs and Patents Act 1988

ISBN 9781800948938

No part of this publication may be reproduced, stored
in a retrieval system, or transmitted, in any form or
by any means, electronic, mechanical, photocopying,
recording or otherwise, without the prior
permission of the publisher

Cover design (AI)
Michael Terence Publishing

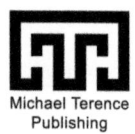

Michael Terence
Publishing

This book is dedicated to our wonderful, brave fathers, and Claire's mother - you left us far too soon. We continue to feel your guidance and love throughout our Cosmic journey, and you will hold a special place in our hearts, forever and always!

We are eternally grateful for the support our husbands have shown us. Your love, support and constant belief in us whilst we worked on our books, astrological research, and our Cosmic app.

And to our beautiful children who make our hearts burst with pride every single day. We did it for you!

We are forever thankful for the support and love we have been shown by family, friends, and clients, who show so much passion and dedication to our method.

Foreword 1
Disclaimer 3
Glossary of Terms 4
Where It All Began 6
Other Sway Methods 8
Dr Eugen Jonas 13
Dr Jonas' LFD Method 15
Luminaries and Our Biological Ovulation 17
The Moon 18
The Eight Phases 19
The New and Full Moon 20
The Zodiacs 24
How the Zodiacs Sway 25
Zodiacs Personal to You 26
Weaker/Stronger Zodiac Signs 28
Groundbreaking Research 30
Void of Course (VOC) 31
Polarity 33
The Human Egg 34
Egg Polarity and Ions 35
Ions and the Moon 38
Ions to Sway Girl 40
Ions to Sway Boy 41
Crystals 42
pH and Why it's Important 45
What Makes Us Different 47
Our Cosmic Girl Sway Method 48
Our Girl Sway Guidelines 50
Our Cosmic Boy Sway Method 51
Our Boy Sway Guidelines 53
Abstinence 54

How to Analyse Ovulation – Ov+8 57
pH 59
pH Test Strips 60
Why Are There So Many Variables? 62
The Biological Side 64
Ovulation 66
Recording LH 69
False Surges 78
Cosmic Peak 80
Tips and Tricks on How to Follow Your Most Fertile Signs 81
Cervical Mucus 83
Types of Cervical Fluids 85
Cervical Position 87
BBT (Basal Body Temperature) 89
Sperm 92
Chemo-attractants 94
Chemo-attractants – They Do Not Determine Your Baby's Gender 96
The Cosmic Sway App 97
The Cosmic Sway Client Page 98
Supplements 99
Folate 102
NAC 104
Myo-Inositol 107
CoQ10 108
Ginger 110
Vitamin D 112
Vitamin E – 400mg 113
Vitamin B12 – 150 mcg 114
Zinc – 50mg 116
Vitex 118

Sex Selection Supplements 120
Boy Sway Extras 123
For Your Partner 128
Girl Sway Lubricants 130
Boy Sway Alkalinity 133
Aiding Implantation 135
Acupuncture to Aid Fertility 144
How can Acupuncture Help Boost Fertility? 145
Natural Fertility 146
Pregnancy Testing and the Two Week Wait 148
Ready to Test? 150
Things to Do in the Two Week Wait 151
Closing 152

Foreword

Together, by combining astrology and science, we've created a sway and fertility enhancing method, using your lunar biorhythmic cycle, your biological ovulation, and the powerful forces of the zodiacs. The Moon has a powerful pull when it comes to creating life.

A regular menstrual cycle, (which regulates fertility), is the same length as the lunar month. Yes, women vary in their cycles, but on average match the 29.5-day lunar cycle. Hard science will say that's just a coincidence. We don't believe this to be true. Once you understand the way life and how the universe really works, the flow of energy, information, and intelligence that directs every moment, then you begin to see the amazing meanings and messages all around you!

By incorporating the research of Dr Eugen Jonas, an astrologist, gynecologist and psychiatrist, along with our 14 years of experience within natural sex selection, gender joy can be yours. Most of us know that the Moon influences the tides, our human behaviours, animals, and the menstrual cycle of women. The lunar cycle has a direct impact on human reproduction, as mentioned above, particularly fertility, menstruation, and birth rates.

The sun's light provides the energy for all living things. But this alone is not enough for life to originate. We must look at helping the biological side of Astro fertility and other proven factors that increase our chances of a viable pregnancy and the gender we desire. The tidal waves show the physical effect of the Moon, she acts as a reflecting body of the sun's light, and due to some possible unknown effect, this is the cause for life to be born.

Without the Moon the Earth would be lifeless. If the Moon is this powerful and plays such a huge role on life, then why wouldn't it be a deciding factor on the sex of your baby? We put our heads together and combined our knowledge of Astro fertility, natural gender selection, spirituality, astronomy and our keen interest in several types of astrology. By using mostly modern Western astrology and crystal healing to enrich our daily lives. Using the Moon's cycles, we open ourselves up to lunar energies and can use her magic to not only live a more fulfilled life but use her divine rhythms for many things.

Pregnancy is a truly magical time for a woman and her partner. This book is intended to not only guide you through our method, every step of the way, but also to explain to you exactly how it works - from understanding how the ions from the zodiacs sway, how egg polarity is the very reason a girl or boy is conceived, and how to track precisely for our method's success to be achieved. We also cover the spiritual element of trying to conceive and how we can give Nature a helping hand.

You'll learn about how to naturally boost fertility and how the conception process comes together. We are looking at every single aspect of our method. We've also handpicked the supplements and other products that we personally use to give you a helping hand and a less stressful experience knowing you're ordering correctly.

Disclaimer

We believe when you are trying to bring new life into the world, it is important to incorporate traditional medicine with spiritual techniques. Always consult with your physician to discuss the ways you can best prepare your body for pregnancy and to rule out any medical issues that may affect your ability to get pregnant. Once you have sought the advice of your doctor, you can proceed with some spiritual and natural methods to help enhance your probability of conceiving.

Natural gender selection increases your odds of having your desired gender - it's no longer 50/50 since the introduction of our amazing, successful method. Our gender selection method relies on conception happening at a precise time. Our bodies aren't robots, and we can have accelerated or delayed ovulation. We can only work on the ovulation predictors available so cannot guarantee that this method achieves 100% success. However, at the time of print our method has reached an <u>incredible 95%</u>.

We are not doctors: Therefore, we advise you to seek medical attention from a healthcare provider before starting your journey.

Glossary of Terms

In this book, and across our social media pages you will come across many acronyms. Here's a list of the most common ones you will see:

AF = Aunt Flo {your period}

BD = Baby Dance {sexual intercourse}

DTD = Doing the Deed {sexual intercourse}

BFP = Big Fat Positive {positive pregnancy test}

BFN = Big Fat Negative {negative positive test}

CD = Cycle Day
{Cycle Day One is the first day of your period}

BBT = Basal Body Temperature

CM = Cervical Mucus

OPK = Ovulation Predictor Kit

CP = Cosmic Peak

CC = Cervical Changes

LH = Luteinizing Hormone

DPO = Days Past Ovulation
{Day One is the day after ovulation}

FMU = First Morning Urine

O = Ovulation

Big O = Orgasm

TTC = Trying to Conceive

HPT = Home Pregnancy Test

2WW = Two Week Wait
{the two weeks from ovulation until your period arrives or a positive pregnancy result}

HCG = Human Chorionic Gonadotropin
{pregnancy hormone}

LFD = Lunar Fertility Day

VOC = Void of Course

PCOS = Polycystic Ovarian Syndrome

EWCM = Egg White Cervical Mucus

Magick = The word Magick is not about cultivating supernatural powers, but rather about aligning oneself with natural forces to manifest an intention.

Where It All Began

We are two mothers that met by chance. Some may use the term coincidence, but we don't believe there's such a thing. When we look at the spiritual laws of the universe, it becomes clear that we're meant to meet everyone who enters our lives. The Law of Divine Oneness explains that every atom, every thought, every action, and every event in the world is inextricably linked with anything and everything else. There's a reason why every person we meet enters our lives - they have something to offer or teach us. And us, them. We were brought together to help each other, and you. You were supposed to find us.

We had both been in the sway world for many years, after we both conceived our sons when trying to sway for baby girls. We searched all avenues to increase our odds of conceiving a girl, we both attempted different sway techniques, and you've guessed it, they were both unsuccessful. Unable to fund several rounds of IVF and having to travel abroad since it's illegal in our country, we found ourselves back at the starting block. With one last chance to fulfil our dreams we knew we had to find the secret formula. And we did. We are very blessed with our sons, which goes without saying. However, we both wanted to experience having little girls of our own. Our little girls are now earthside - thanks to our method.

Gender disappointment is a taboo subject, and it doesn't have to be. We get to live on Mother Earth just once in this body, so enjoying that time and being happy should carry no guilt. Let's be open and honest here, whilst many people won't admit to feelings of disappointment with the gender of their baby, it can be a perfectly normal reaction that's much more common than you've been led to believe.

After many years of research and looking over various sway techniques available on the internet, we were able to debunk several popular sway methods that have been around for a while.

Other Sway Methods

There are several methods available online, many of which boast a high success rate, but do they genuinely deliver those results? Social media has become incredibly influential, particularly for businesses. In the past, women had to rely solely on information from books and trust the claimed success rates before the rise of social media. Now you can view Facebook groups that specifically focus on gender swaying, or the methods we discuss below. There, you can find actual real-life success stories, and non-successful ones.

Let's look at some of these methods and the flaws behind them. We won't add names for the methods described below for legal purposes. We also aren't here to speak derogatorily about other methods either; we simply want to explain our views on why those below aren't quite what some were led to believe.

A popular method from the 1960s that was publicised in a book. Provides an outdated guide on how and when to have intercourse to determine the sex of a foetus. According to the hypothesis, male (Y) sperm are faster but more fragile than female (X) sperm. Further, acidic environments harm Y sperm, according to the theory, making conception of a girl more likely. This method aims to exploit these two factors.

They concluded that the larger-headed sperms were that of the XX and the smaller-headed sperms were that of the XY. They began to perform and publish studies based on this idea, write books, and still to this date their findings have been left as gospel. The issue is, Dr Shettles was wrong with his findings (confirmed by scientists today). What he was really looking at was 'capacitated' and 'uncapacitated' sperm. The capacitation process had not yet been discovered when this theory was developed in his timing methodology.

Capacitated sperm are sperm that have lost their protective caps, which means they're ready to fertilise an egg. They moved faster and so this was wrongfully thought to be XY sperm. Uncapacitated sperm were bigger and slower because they were still wearing their protective caps, (unable to fertilise the egg) and so they were wrongfully thought to be XX sperm.

Eventually, when uncapacitated sperm lose their protective cap, they will all be the same size and move at the same speed, but they will both be the X and Y sperm, whether they have a cap or whether they don't. Sperm capacitates in waves, and they seem to be able to communicate with each other on some primitive level to coordinate this process, so if there are living sperm present, some will be capacitated and ready to fertilize the egg. Over the course of time, the capacitated sperm die - capacitated sperm don't live too long after they lose their caps, So, when Dr Shettles makes the claim that "Y sperm don't live as long", what he was really observing was the early deaths of capacitated sperm. Capacitated sperm dies sooner than incapacitated sperm, but X and Y sperm live the same length of time.

Another known method which was completely derived from a previous theory "the Billings method" - the method which was studied on cows! You heard it, the study was also done on humans which resulted in a 60% success rate, unfortunately this was never written in the book.

So, what was the study? The study which was based on cows saw them inseminate several cows 2-3 days before ovulation (or so-called ovulation). They based this on the cow's behaviour and their cervical mucus; to have a boy calf they inseminated the cow 24 hours and 48 hours after predicted ovulation and to have a girl calf they would inseminate the cow 2-3 days before predicted ovulation.

We believe the flaw in this is apparent - you cannot clearly identify ovulation by looking at cervical mucus, or your overall behaviour. Yes, cervical mucus changes as we hit our fertile days, but not all cervical patterns are the same, so this isn't dependable at all and who knows when the cow conceived without proper ovulation confirmation?

The book goes on further to state their method is as easy as tracking ovulation and nothing else is needed to sway. However, we know that science has confirmed that other factors help. This method also has its very own Facebook group which a few years ago tracked results. Unfortunately, the failed sways became so high they no longer kept track. More recently a high profile celebrity tried this method and is having her first girl after having four boys. Coincidentally, the method wasn't entirely followed to plan, and she did the opposite of what the book says to do for a girl. We believe the failed sways are down to the timing method used for her sway, the attempts before ovulation for a girl are when the body is at its most alkaline, and the attempts after ovulation for a boy is when the reproductive tract is now acidic, which favours female sperm and is a likely reason for failed boy sways.

A third method, which employed a similar concept to ours, but relied solely on the zodiacs for gender swaying. However, we follow the facts and science around how Astro fertility works, alongside our biological ovulation, which is why our success rate is much higher.

There were multiple, concerning errors with this method before the founder of the method left her Facebook groups and her clients behind her, her success rate sitting at 53%. So where did it all go wrong? Confusion and misinformation. Not taking pH into account, allowing women to attempt multiple times during their surge, in a 48-hour window.

We know pH is one of the main factors as to how a baby boy or baby girl is conceived. Multiple attempts will increase the vaginal fluids, reaching levels of up to 14 (highly alkaline), as well the follicle fluid surrounding our biological egg and therefore altering the egg's outer shell. If your pH is not at the correct levels, then the opposite sex will be conceived. Egg polarity is key to gender swaying, and when the pH levels are too high, the egg polarity will be polarised for a male bearing sperm. Finally, the biological side of ovulation. To have success using the Zodiacs to sway, you must time intercourse perfectly. Conception must occur in the correct Zodiac phase for you. And if you don't track ovulation or basal body temperature correctly, then we can't be sure where conception occurs.

They believed ovulation occurred 12 hours after a peak OPK. Our data proved otherwise, not only from our clients but also scientific research. In fact, the average is between 24-28 hours. We have many ladies that ovulate after 24 hours and some that are at the end of the scale at 40 hours. The most common we've noted in our group is 28. Though we don't ignore the broad spectrum. We also know that the Zodiacs are individual to us and our birth charts (we will go into this in more detail later). It simply isn't as easy as conceiving in a female sign, and a baby girl is conceived, or vice versa. If it were that simple, there would no longer be any need for IVF sex selection.

Dr Eugen Jonas

We've mentioned him briefly, now let's look at where this all links in with our method. The Lunar Fertility Method dates back to ancient Babylonia, in which an ancient manuscript said that a woman's fertility was based on the Moon. However, for years, this concept remained relatively obscure.

It was Dr Jonas who unearthed the manuscript and decided in 1956 to test this theory on women. He eventually opened a fertility clinic in Czechoslovakia, but it was closed by the Communist regime. We spent a large amount of time researching Dr Eugen Jonas and his brilliant work. When he found that women can have an extra, secondary ovulation each month (your Lunar Fertile Day!) he changed many women's lives. During the time when the angle of the Sun and the Moon occur at the exact same time of your own birth, you may release another egg, and this egg will already be polarised for a certain sex.

How, you ask? Jonas found that the sex of the offspring is related to certain phases of the Moon at the time of conception. The astrological sign in which the Moon is at, at the time of one's own conception, should be decisive over the gender of the child. It all began from an assertion in an Assyrian source that Jonas happened to find in a library: "Woman is fertile during a certain phase of the Moon." But which phase exactly? After a lengthy period of research and endless calculations, he managed to find the answer. He wrote: "Finally, on August 15, 1956, I arrived at the first three fundamental rules on conception, the determination of sex and life capability of the foetus, all of which can be precisely formulated."

In the summer of 1956, Dr Jonas made an extensive trial, testing over 10,000 women. Comparing conception charts, he searched for a pattern. After testing and researching in the fields of astronomy and astrology, Dr Jonas observed a correlation between the Moon activity and fertility cycles. He discovered that under certain circumstances a woman's fertility is subject to periodic variations which have an influence on conception as well as conceiving a baby of specific sex. With a group of Cosmo biologists, Jonas discovered three fundamental rules on conception, the sex determination, and the viability of the foetus.

Dr Jonas' LFD Method

Dr Jonas' method was based on a separate spontaneous ovulation that can occur once a month when the Sun and Moon are at the same angle as they were at the time of your birth. We know from our own studies that this occurs around 15-20% of the time. But for Jonas it worked 85% of the time, so why is it different now? We have things like Wi-Fi, medication, supplements, chemicals, more positive ions in the air. All these things have likely affected the triggering of our spontaneous ovulation. We also know that a lot of the women from Dr Jonas' studies fell pregnant when they were on their Aunt Flow. Combine that with an orgasm, and the triggering of their spontaneous ovulation happened. From his stats it was happening a lot.

His success rate was 98% for sex selection, which is incredible. However, applying the same method alongside your biological ovulation wasn't. We saw this mistake from another group. Jonas himself warned about combining the two, he gave a percentage of 87% when they both coincide, but we can now confirm it's a lot lower. His graphs would cross out the days around ovulation, so intercourse wasn't allowed 7 days before and 7 days after (sperm survival). Then he would have you attempt for 3 days leading up to your Lunar Fertile Day (even on AF) in the hope you trigger your LFD egg and conceive in the time frame given.

You can find your LFD day either by downloading our app or searching your "lunar fertile return" on the web. Astro-seek is a great website and very useful. LFD is based on the Sun and Moon at the time you were born (you see it's all based on us, as individuals). When each month the Sun and Moon angle is in a male or female Zodiac, you will conceive either a girl or a boy.

Now, here's the tricky part, most of the time you won't see an LH surge with your spontaneous egg, so you won't get the build-up of pH in your reproductive tract. The egg released for LFD is already polarised and ready for a female or male bearing sperm. The LFD egg will only release within that two-hour window given, and sperm will already be waiting for the egg, so conception will 100% happen inside the female or male phase.

He had a very specific and reliable formulation for his LFD. This didn't just include the Sun and Moon; therefore, he knew that if the egg was triggered at that exact point the energies, and other alignments, would produce the preferred sex of the child. Notice how he also recognized the change in pH in the reproductive tract at varying times of your fertility cycle.

Luminaries and Our Biological Ovulation

The mistake that, well, we all made really, was believing that LFD and bio-O combined would be a golden sway. Sadly, after our second LFD and bio-O failure we had to dive deeper into the astrology side and work out why it wasn't yielding the same results.

It really didn't take us long to see why he advised against it. Of course, the science around bio-o mattered, he said it himself. When the Moon floated through the different signs of the Zodiacs the womb sedimentation changed, thus altering the egg polarity to conceive a boy or girl. So, LFD was a separate egg - you likely won't get an LH surge as it's completely spontaneous. Bio-logical ovulation isn't, therefore when combining the two, add in the pH side, also not to mention where your bio-logical egg will drop, and where conception may even take place, plus the cosmos influences. It becomes extremely risky!

We know that your LFD is a two-hour window only, (confirmed by an astrologist herself!) and conception must occur in that two-hour window. That's slim, the likelihood of your biological ovulation falling in that two-hour window is, well, not only risky, but around 5%, let's say. So, for that reason we advise solo swayers against it. However, with our expert help and our own cosmic calculation, we can now guide you on a specific LFD and bio-logical ovulation sway.

The Moon

Let's look at some evidence-based facts and you'll see why we believe so strongly in the power of the Moon. The Moon is Earth's only natural satellite and causes the tides to rise and fall, but we have discovered many more amazing facts about that astronomical body.

The Moon changes its apparent shape with four distinct phases depending on the Moon's position as it orbits around the Earth, and the Earth's position as it orbits around the Sun. There are four main Moon phases, also known as Lunar Phases: First Quarter, Full Moon, Last Quarter and New Moon. An additional four intermediate phases make up the combined eight phases that comprise the Phases of the Moon in the following sequential order: New Moon, Waxing Crescent, First Quarter, Waxing Gibbous, Full Moon, Waning Gibbous, Last Quarter and Waning Crescent.

The Eight Phases

The Moon displays these eight phases one after the other as it moves through its cycle each month. It takes 27 days for the Moon to orbit Earth, which means the Moon's cycle is 27 days long. Traditionally the female cycle is known as the "Moon Cycle".

a) The menstrual cycle follows the lunar cycle – between 28-31 days;

b) Menstruation occurs at a New Moon and;

c) It has a say over our libido and sex life. The Moon is part of a rhythm observed in the natural world of cycles, with Life Force developing, growing, and energising during the waxing cycle (up to the Full Moon), and reducing during the waning cycle (Full Moon - New Moon).

The New and Full Moon

The New Moon is when the Sun and Moon are aligned, with the Sun and Earth on opposite sides of the Moon. At New Moon, the Sun, the Moon, and Earth are in alignment. The New Moon is the first lunar phase, occurring when both the Sun and the Moon have the same ecliptic longitude.

During the New Moon phase, the lunar disk is invisible to the naked eye, except when it is silhouetted during a solar eclipse. For many decades, the New Moon term was used to describe the first visible crescent of the Moon after its conjunction with the Sun. A New Moon, in astronomy, marks the beginning of the first lunar phase. Many believe that this symbolises new beginnings, and some people even start new projects during this lunar phase, feeling that the Moon's energy will favour them. For humans, the New Moon is a time to rest and to recharge the batteries, as the Moon is doing the same thing. At this time, the Moon blends with the darkness of the night for a brief time, only to come back to life with new forces. All around the world, cycles are most likely to start around the time of the full Moon when night skies are brightest. On the flipside, a woman will be most fertile with the New Moon - when it is barely visible. The perfect time to set intentions, whereas the Full Moon is the time to reap the rewards. On each New Moon you say cheerio to the last phase and welcome the fresh one with renewed energy.

The same principle applies if you are doing a Full Moon ritual. We cover more on this in our manifestation book, and there is no right or wrong, we do what works best for us and gives us a feeling of being calm and centred, which can only help the process of conception taking place. Manifestation is setting your intention for something you want to happen and then witnessing it happen in the real world. In other words, if you believe it, it will happen. The "law of attraction," or the belief that you get whatever you send out into the universe, underpins manifestation. When we manifest, we are pulling up energy from the earth to bring it to form. Remember your power.

As the Full Moon is associated with fertility, it is a good time for cultivating and nourishing femininity. Apart from that, this phase of the Moon allows for heightened creativity, innovative breakthroughs, and reconnecting with your intuition. Performing a full Moon manifestation or ritual can help with transforming into your highest self.

Have you ever heard of people saying they're collecting Moon water and wondered what that is and what they're doing with it? We are those people collecting Moon water. We love doing this. We will also leave some of our crystals out that evening in the garden to recharge under the power of the Full Moon and allow them to soak in the moonlight. Please be mindful that certain types of crystals cannot be exposed to water and can get damaged. The ritual does not need to be completed at the exact moment of a Full Moon but should be performed within 48 hours before or after for best results. You can do as much or as little as you want, follow your intuition and allow this to guide you.

One of the oldest and most powerful fertility enhancement techniques is a ritual bath. Ritual bathing involves using special herbs to impart essences that are conducive to achieving your desired goal - in this case, conception. Spiritual baths have the multi-faceted effects of relaxation of the body and stimulation of the inner self. A time to unwind, manifest and take care of yourself. Add some bath salts, our favourite is lavender essential oil and Epsom salts, but you may prefer an uplifting sweet orange or lemon.

In ancient times, a woman's cycle was honoured and celebrated - how amazing this is. While her bleeding phase was ritualised. Women of all ages came together in sacred circles and moon lodges. Getting your moon period was seen as a beautiful gift. It was a blessing and a celebration. Bleeding would be a time for resting, journeying inwards, and tuning in to your intuition - letting go of anything that no longer served you, resetting, and starting afresh.

But the Patriarchy felt threatened by the power and magick that these women held within, which only magnified their force when they came together. So what was once seen as beautiful and pure became stigmatised and seen as taboo, much like gender swaying and gender disappointment.

It doesn't have to be that way. We don't have to see our period as a hassle, a burden, and sometimes even a curse. She stands for all that is us, we are blessed, and the feminine energy is transforming. We are awakening to the Lunar energies and who we are as women.

In terms of fertility, the Moon is the most important planet for both men and women. The Moon rules the entire reproductive process, but reproduction is such a huge and essential function of every species, that all the planets have some involvement and influence. We find it comforting to look at the night sky and remember that hundreds of cultures and billions of people have seen the same stars and Moon.

The Zodiacs

All Zodiac signs are divided into two sets of dualities, which are known as polarities. Like elements and modalities, which refer to what drives each sign and how they contribute to the world, polarities are another way of categorising Zodiac signs. If you look at the Zodiac wheel, you'll notice that the dualities switch off every other sign, which illustrates the ebb and flow of certain energies as planets travel through the Zodiac. This also means that the adjacent signs to any Zodiac sign will always be of the opposite duality, while the opposing sign on the Zodiac wheel will be the same. Each Zodiac sign is thought to have "positive" or "negative" charge to its energy (ions), which are also described as being active versus receptive. Yin and Yang.

How the Zodiacs Sway

We incorporated the Zodiacs into our method because their polarity is what will help strengthen your sway. Negative ions - sway <u>girl</u> and positive ions - sway <u>boy</u>. Ions will alter the charge to your biological egg's polarity.

The Zodiacs also have their own polarity based on you, and your birth chart. This will increase the odds for a higher success. When we ovulate, our eggs sit in a follicular fluid, this fluid will also have its own pH polarity, too.

Do you see where we're going with polarity being the focus? Each Zodiac sign is thought to have a "positive" or "negative" charge to its energy, also described as being active versus receptive. For a long time, the two dualities were known primarily as "masculine" and "feminine" energies. The membrane of each sperm will also carry a positive or negative charge. If the sperm and egg have the same charge at the time of meeting they will repel, and the egg won't be fertilised. If they are both opposite, <u>they will be attracted to each other</u>.

Zodiacs Personal to You

After hundreds of sways, we were able to identify a pattern that blew our minds. It made sense, when you look at our luminaires and how the expert himself identified this spontaneous ovulation. It soon became apparent to us - this was based on us, as individuals.

When we opened our Cosmic Sway FB group in 2021.We always knew there was more to the Zodiacs, and by incorporating all things scientific, alongside the Zodiacs, our group was soon flooded with successes. Some mantras stick with people, like timing for example or the use of the zodiacs to sway alone. And our method is completely different, but it took time for people to see that our timing methodology was successful and there most certainly is more to the zodiacs than we all initially believed.

We were soon sat at a 90% success rate, and we were over the moon. Yet we wanted to strive for more. We gave ourselves a goal, a 95% success rate and to give as many ladies as we could gender joy. And guess what, we did it!

So how are the Zodiacs personal to us? Just like our luminaries (LFD), the exact moment we are born we have our own birth print, the same as our fingerprints, no one will ever have the same. Our birth print is ours, it's a snapshot of the sky at the very moment you took your first breath, it's when you come into specific energies of the universe, which then remain fixed throughout your entire lifetime.

The Cosmic Sway Method

Throughout our three and a half years of dedicated research and being lucky enough to have a huge range of data to analyse, we found some groundbreaking evidence that really excited us. We've been so close to finding the missing piece to the puzzle, and after adding all the variables and finding the last piece, our cosmic formula was created. Much like Jonas and his LFD formula, we now have ours. We were able to find a correlation between your natal charts and natural sex selection. At first it seemed coincidental, but the more we looked, the more these patterns lined up. This means that for natural sex selection, your stronger Zodiacs will have a stronger pull to your ovum's polarity.

Weaker/Stronger Zodiac Signs

It's true! Even astrologers will agree. Our birth charts hold a wealth of information! They reveal insights into our personality traits, help us understand ourselves more deeply, and illuminate our desires and connections to the universe. Additionally, the zodiacs in your natal chart can play a huge role in natural sex selection. Humans are part of a vast cosmic tapestry that includes celestial entities like planets, stars, moons, and asteroids.

Some suggest that our connection to the celestial realms goes beyond mere geographic location. For instance, many elements in our bodies were formed in stars billions of years ago. Isn't that fascinating? Your natal chart contains significant insights about the energies present at the exact moment of your birth. On a personal level, it highlights your strengths and weaknesses, indicating the best and worst times to undertake major life changes. The primary reason understanding your natal chart is so important is that it is uniquely yours.

We first noticed the Zodiacs weren't quite what they seemed rather quickly. We had received quite a few emails from ladies with failed sways, from numerous other pages, and after a full four weeks of investigating, we found a very similar pattern with two Zodiacs. It was almost like they had switched genders! Leo became favourable for a girl sway, and Pisces became favourable for a boy sway. The pattern was clear, ladies with multiples of the same sex couldn't sway inside those specific zodiacs. But why?

We kept digging! At this point, we felt like Jonas himself, with hundreds of ladies' sway data, we found many astrological patterns. We printed every single one of them out alongside their natal charts. We started highlighting, drawing lines everywhere, writing notes down, and there was the lightbulb moment. We had made the connection. Our minds were blown. Right there we knew the Zodiacs absolutely do sway, 100% they do.

However, and this is fact, it isn't that every female sign will mean you will conceive a baby girl, or every male sign will mean you will conceive a baby boy, not for biological ovulation anyway. There will be Zodiacs that will be stronger for you to sway in, and some that will be weaker. Only a birth chart analysis will identify which signs are stronger or weaker for you to sway in.

And drum roll please… you will be able to sway inside a weaker male zodiac and conceive a baby GIRL or vice versa. Simply put, our personal zodiacs polarise differently to the phases you can sway in. At the time of print we have helped six clients sway inside a male zodiac, all six have confirmed their babies to be girls. How? We analysed their birth charts and identified which Zodiacs were their strongest and weakest. You can find these results via our Facebook group.

Groundbreaking Research

We were thrilled to discover some groundbreaking astrological insights related to natural sex selection. It took us three-and-a-half years of daily immersion in birth charts and data to unravel these findings. We identified seven key elements that, when combined, ensure a remarkable 98% success rate for the gender you are hoping to sway.

This is not merely the singular day that was noted long ago regarding spontaneous ovulation. In February 2024, we found that conceiving in your Moon sign provides the strongest Zodiac influence for swaying, while conceiving in your Sun sign only aligns for 65% of the gender you are aiming for.

However, as we've noted, the situation isn't as straightforward as that. External factors can significantly affect these outcomes. We're considering multiple celestial influences, and everything must align perfectly for the most effective sway. We are excited to share the Moon and Sun variables, as we believe this will benefit those swaying alone; this information is vital and has never been disclosed until now. However, we cannot reveal the complete calculations or the factors that can override these variables. The Zodiac alone is not everything, but this is groundbreaking information brought to you by us - the Cosmic Sway Method.

Void of Course (VOC)

The Moon will change signs every 40-48 hours - and this is where precision in tracking your ovulation, and our expertise is crucial. VOC will occur multiple times a week and the duration ranges from 24 to two hours. VOC happens when the Moon is making its final major aspect with another planet before changing signs.

The Moon moves so quickly through the Zodiacs, it is the fastest-moving planet in astrology after all. The Moon is constantly forming aspects with other planets which is what causes the effects on our moods and. all other energies around us. The planets ignite her power, but she's always floating through the Zodiac and only at the point of VOC does the Moon float through the Zodiac without any influence from the other planets that are usually there to bounce their energy off her.

So, we know this does not mean the Moon is never completely alone from the Zodiacs. This, unfortunately, was a mistake made by other methods. The founder of the group believed that this space in time meant the Moon was completely alone thus meaning if you fell into that period your sway would be 50/50 since there was no Zodiac accompanying the Moon at that time. The fact is, the Moon will always be in a sign and void of course is where the Moon has already made all the aspects it will make whilst in that sign. The Moon won't make another aspect until it enters a new sign. Therefore, the Zodiacs will run from one to another. Once one phase ends it will enter a new phase and Zodiac. There is no period where the gender is neutral as the Moon will always be in a male or female Zodiac. In simple terms, the Void of Course Moon describes the period before the Moon moves into a new sign during which it doesn't form any significant meet ups with any of the other planets. You can feel the switch of those signs.

Polarity

Polarity in astrology is one of the classifications which the Zodiac signs are grouped into - specifically, in astrology, polarity refers to the energetic charge or orientation of a planet or Zodiac sign. Every planet and Zodiac sign in astrology is assigned either a positive or negative polarity. This designation is not a value judgement, but rather a way of categorising the unique energy of each celestial body. Every part of our sway's focus is about polarity! The Zodiac, sperm and the ovum. They all count.

It's been proven that depending on whether sperm carry an X or Y chromosome, spermatozoa have opposite polarisation. The X spermatozoa have a negative charge, and the Y spermatozoa have a positive charge. This was observed when the X and Y spermatozoa were separated by electrophoresis. Numerous studies revealed that when a weak electrical current was passed through a solution containing spermatozoa, those with the X chromosome were attracted by the anode (+) and those with the Y chromosome by the cathode (−). Scientists at the university of Roscoff also identified the appearance of a brief luminous ring of contact between spermatozoon and ovule. This phenomenon has been measured and is proof of an electrical polarisation at the exact point of fertilisation.

The Human Egg

The membrane surrounding a human egg also emits ions, transmitting an electrical "charge" of its own. It is this energy that attracts either the X or Y sperm. This is why the Zodiacs sway. We've been so excited to share this.

Depending on whether sperm is carrying an X or Y chromosome, there will be an opposite polarisation. The X spermatozoa have a negative charge, and the Y spermatozoa have a positive charge. Studies have been carried out to prove this - there's an electrical involvement in fertilisation and the connection is the positive and negative charge from the Zodiacs (your most favourable) when egg and sperm meet.

Egg Polarity and Ions

The male body has one polarity and the female the other. To the male, his polarity feels positive, and to the female, her polarity feels negative. When they unite sexually, they can each sense a completeness that occurs when both polarities are felt simultaneously. Whether the controlling factor of the Moon over the menstrual cycle is the gravitational pull, the increase in light, the ionisation of the atmosphere, the changes in electromagnetic conditions or, more probably, a combination of all of these and perhaps other effects, is not known, but as the ancients and primitive peoples in touch with nature have all known, and as Science is finding out, this connection is obvious and undeniable.

Ions are believed to affect the egg's polarity and pH levels. Positive and negative ions come from many different sources, and some people are more affected by them than others. As we've discussed, Y sperm are positively charged, and high in pH. At different stages our cervical mucus will switch and become negatively charged to positively charged. When negatively charged, you need a negatively charged egg to attract a positively charged Y sperm. Positive sways boy, negative for a girl.

Here's how it works: ions are constantly giving and taking because opposites attract. The polarity of the ovum membrane is not fixed but alternates from positive to neutral to negative. This is called the Polarity Cycle. You can control this cycle with ions and lubricant, so if you're swaying for a boy increasing your alkalinity in your cervical mucus can help. Attempt prior to ovulation when the reproductive tract is more alkaline. And when you're in your favourable Zodiac your mucus will be at the right molecular level to attract the XY sperm. The Y sperm will become positively charged when they enter a high pH (this makes them stronger), and swim at a faster rate, causing the XY sperm to move faster toward the egg. When the spermatozoa reach the egg, the polarity will be the right environment as your cervical mucus pH. The negative egg then attracts the Y-bearing sperm. High pH in your CM creates more negative ions (we know this sounds a little crazy, and somewhat confusing!) So, when we expose ourselves to positive ions, that makes the egg negative which causes the CM to have negative ions, thus a higher pH. This happens because there is a give-and-take effect. Ions are always trading to balance (this is kind of like when you drink lemon juice - It's acidic until it enters your body and turns alkaline). This is because the polarity of the ovum is not fixed, it can be bumped into the correct polarity by using the opposite ions desired.

To recap: Positive ions make the egg negative because of the alternating nature of the polarity of the ovum and because ions are always trying to balance themselves. CM reacts by becoming negative (negative ions means high pH) The egg is full of negative ions thus attracting the XY sperm.

Ions are believed to affect the egg's polarity and pH levels. Positive and negative ions come from many different sources, and some people are more affected by them than others. Ions are molecules that have gained or lost an electron through various atmospheric forces or environmental influences. They are created in nature by the effects of water, air, radiation, and sunlight. Often nicknamed as "vitamin in air", an ion can help to improve body growth and prevent diseases. We believe they have an influence when we put everything together.

It's another factor that points to how the universe works in tandem with human beings. Astrology is a science, after all, so why wouldn't the ions that we surround ourselves with daily, link? You may hear people mention when swaying girl that they used "lavender everything" and surrounded themselves with salt lamps and fans. This is why.

Ions and the Moon

It seems that the Moon affects natural phenomena in four main ways:

Firstly, through its gravitational pull on fluids and, secondly, by the changing amount of light it shines on the Earth. The third effect is less well known, but it appears that the Moon influences atmospheric ionisation, the electrical charging of atoms. Positive ions, which, for example, build up prior to a storm, are notorious for their deleterious effect on mental and physical health, causing a stuffy headache and faint feeling of listlessness and feeling uneasy. Negative ions, as generated by ionisers and which are prevalent after a storm or near the sea, cause a feeling of physical and psychological well-being. A Full Moon is supposed to bring an increase in positive ions, and the negative ions increase as the Moon wanes.

From weeping trees to teeth stronger than Kevlar, senior curator Dr Tom White sheds some light on a few of the fascinating, unnoticed ways the Moon shapes the course of life on Earth. "The Moon has been up there as long as evolution has been taking place, and lunar rhythms are embedded in the life cycles of many organisms. The challenge is working out when the Moon truly is a factor and what is merely myth and legend."

According to Tom, there are three main ways in which the Moon impacts on life: time, tides, and light. "For many animals, particularly birds, the Moon is essential to migration and navigation. Others will time their reproduction to coincide with the specific phases of the lunar cycle. There is also a whole world of fascinating adaptations relating to tides and the unique properties of moonlight."

Ions to Sway Girl

Negative ions exist in nature in tons of places, including ultraviolet (UV) rays from the Sun, discharges of electricity in the air after a thunderclap or lightning strike, wherever water collides with itself like a waterfall, or the ocean shore (creating the Lennard-Jones Potential - produced as part of the normal growth process for many plants.)

Negative ions are odourless, tasteless, and invisible molecules that we inhale in abundance in certain environments. Think mountains, waterfalls, and beaches and of course the Zodiac phases. Once they reach our bloodstream, negative ions are believed to produce biochemical reactions that increase levels of the mood chemical serotonin, helping to alleviate depression, relieve stress, and boost our daytime energy.

Ions to Sway Boy

Positive ions. Positive ions make the egg negative CM react by becoming negative ions (negative ions means high pH). Y sperm love high pH (that's what they are), however, they are attracted to negative ions. The egg is full of negative ions thus attracting the Y sperm.

A scientist named Dr Patrick Schoun, and some others, have suggested that negative ions help sway gender towards girls, and positive ions towards boys. When an atom gains electrons, this results in a negative charge. This type of ion is called an anion. When an atom loses electrons, this results in a positive charge. A positively charged ion is called a cation. Enjoy exploring several examples of ions of both types. Positive ions are typically metals or act like metals; phones, Wi-Fi, laptops, male Zodiacs. Positive ions are more often found in environments that have artificial lighting and a small amount of airflow.

Crystals

Yes, crystals sway too, they are ions! The magick of crystal healing has been used since ancient Egyptian times. It's an amazing alternative therapy to aid conception. And you can also select crystals that have a feminine or masculine energy.

Crystals enrich our lives in many ways: by calming the body and mind, fixing hormonal imbalances, and reducing levels of stress. Crystals for fertility help increase the chances of pregnancy, also. Healing crystals emit delicate energy that boosts your vitality, and eventually, your fertility. Crystals used for fertility have their own frequency, dependent on the element arrangement within their chemical composition. Every element vibrates at a particular frequency, pretty much the way we do, and subtle healing energy is released by this vibration.

The energies emitted by crystals rely on the special way their components vibrate in the inner crystalline structure. It is known that when crystals are held close to the body, the human electromagnetic field changes. While healing occurs, crystals absorb the body's negative energies and release positive energy that the body absorbs throughout the healing process, producing energy-level equilibrium.

You can charge your crystals under the Moon anytime you need answers or a little spiritual boost or pick-me-up. Whether you wear them as jewellery, keep them beside your bed, or have a few in your purse, your crystals will help you on your gender sway journey - all you have to do is hold your crystal, and say your intentions and they will represent what it is you want to achieve, a son or a daughter. They will act as your visual reminder and will be with you on your journey to motherhood.

Discover additional ways to tap into your Lunar Energies with our upcoming spiritual book. This insightful guide delves deeper into the spiritual facets of our approach, featuring topics such as spirit baby connections and manifestation. It explores spiritual themes and spirit baby communications, and emphasises holistic practices, metaphysics, and manifestation, including elements of magic and lunar energy.

Girl Swayers
For girl swayers, we recommend amethyst. Though not a fertility-specific crystal, amethyst is a natural tranquilliser, stress reliever, soothes irritability, balances mood swings, dispels anger, rage, fear, and anxiety. It alleviates sadness and grief, and dissolves negativity and also holds a feminine energy. Like the rose quartz - which is our second choice - as this helps you channel your divine feminine energy.

Boy Swayers
Crystals to harness masculine energy. These are the best crystals to tap into the divine masculine auras around you. The first two we have worked with more and find them to be super powerful: Black Tourmaline - a negative energy protector, it shields you from unwanted energy, like a bodyguard; it is strong and has a manly aura. Tigers Eye Fierce - courageous, bringing you bold, brave energy.

Cleansing and Charging our Crystals

They look beautiful just as they are; to work with our crystals and tap into their energy intended to benefit us, you must cleanse and charge them when you first receive them. They have travelled before they reached you and they are absorbing the energy that is around them. Even down to the postman that handled and delivered them to you! They will absorb the energy they come into contact with, and you want to remove all of that so it is back to its natural form ready to work as it should for you.

If your crystals are on a necklace/bracelet etc. and you are wearing them daily, you can cleanse them when you get them home, or weekly. For those that remain in your home it is not necessary to cleanse as often. As soon as we handle new crystals, we clear all energies, either using sage, selenite, the Moon or Palo Santo. The choice is yours; you may choose to use multiple cleansing properties.

pH and Why it's Important

We often hear: "My vaginal pH is a 4, so I'm good! Many women do not understand that our pH will vary during our cycle. Your vaginal pH will likely always be on the lower side until around ovulation. You see, we need follicle fluid to get super alkaline to protect the sperm and encourage fertilisation.

The female reproductive tract has its own unique pH environment, which changes throughout the menstrual cycle. During ovulation, the cervical mucus becomes more alkaline, creating a favourable environment for sperm survival and motility. Vaginal pH strips will likely test low, but this isn't a true reflection of how high our follicle fluid will become. The follicle fluid that sits around the ovum will reach levels of between 7 to 14, this is fact!

Alkaline pH and Acidic pH: Numerous studies confirm this, including Jonas himself, who believed that as the Moon passed through the different signs of the Zodiacs during your luminaries, the alkalinity of the womb became acidic/alkaline affecting the sedimentation of the sperm. Obviously, this goes against what we're saying, well, the first part anyway.

We can tell what you're thinking - do I need to be alkaline or acidic? What we're explaining here is the process of our pH and the changes it goes through and why it's important for those not trying to sway the odds and simply wanting to get pregnant. Further on you'll see where we explain our timing methodology and why this is important to swaying and how pH comes into play.

What Makes Us Different

Research - and plenty of it. Now you've seen the evidence and science behind our method, we can now look at how Cosmic was created. Over the years, we've studied, worked, and thrown ourselves into the world of astrology, astronomy and fertility. We've spent a large amount of time researching Dr Eugen Jonas and his hugely successful Lunar Fertile Day method.

As previously mentioned, your Lunar Fertile Day is a spontaneous ovulation that occurs each month around the time you were born. The time of the highest woman's fertility coincides with the recurrence of the angle of the Sun and the Moon that occurred at the woman's own birth. This is why we knew we had to dig deeper.

If our spontaneous egg is released at the exact time of one's birth, and that can guarantee a 98% success for your preferred sex, then we had to find the answer to our bio-logical ovulation. Although not 98%, we're proud of our results. It is much more complex than having sex/or ovulating in a female Zodiac and that will guarantee a girl, or vice versa. IVF clinics all over the world would be out of business if it was that simple! Science is what counts and when you combine the evidence we've compiled, we have our perfect bio-ovulation sway.

Our Cosmic Girl Sway Method

Knowing the effects pH has on our egg polarity and reproductive tract during the time of our surge/ovulation, whilst also aligning the ions from the Zodiacs, the chances of the gender you'll likely conceive will be female.

The timing of intercourse in relation to ovulation does matter - the pH level in the reproductive tract (not vagina) is what sways. Negative and positive ions can alter and change our ovum's polarity. The reproductive fluid that sits around your ovum can switch between negative, neutral, and positive. Incorporating the Zodiacs can help keep the egg's polarity negatively charged, favouring a female sperm.

Our very own timing method was also created through years of in-house studies. From the very moment we formulated Cosmic we knew our timing method had to be implemented. Having watched other groups advise ladies to BD multiple times inside a female phase and seeing this result in a 53% success rate, we knew what needed to be done. Having used O+12 to conceive our daughters, and previously spending a large amount of time researching the science behind this, we were confident there was something in it. Although there isn't much to find except one small study. It very much made sense to us!

We've already explained what happens during your surge, however, we haven't explained what happens after. Once we've ovulated, we have a surge in estrogen. This estrogen creates a creamy, lotion-like covering inside our reproductive tract, which becomes acidic. This then creates a perfect environment to conceive a girl. The success rate for this, in over hundreds of women, has been astonishing. We've had two failures in over 400 successes using our girl sway timing. We must state that it can take a little longer to get pregnant, as we want ovulation to happen before it is attempted, however we feel this is worth it when you have results like these.

For O+12 it's important for ladies to understand their bodies, and to have some idea of where ovulation occurs. We started advising our ladies on some tips and tricks to help, and we also advised them to attempt 36 hours after peak. If conception didn't occur, the timing should then be brought down by an hour each month. We noticed pregnancies were mostly occurring between 32-26 hours after peak and so Ov+8 was created!!

We must be mindful that our bodies are not robots. We won't get to 1pm each month and our eggs decide it's time to break through that follicle. Conception after ovulation is key! One month you may ovulate 26 hours after peak, and the following month it may be 34. We won't know for certainty when we ovulate, so looking at all your fertile signs is important.

Our Girl Sway Guidelines

STEP ONE – 5-10 DAY ABSTAIN (DEPENDANT ON PARTNER'S AGE)

STEP TWO – TEST OPKS UNTIL COSMIC PEAK IS REACHED

STEP THREE – CHECK YOUR ZODIACS

STEP FOUR – USE PH-LOWERING LUBRICANTS ONE HOUR BEFORE ATTEMPT

STEP FIVE – CHECK FERTILITY SIGNS, CERVICAL POSITION & CM

STEP SIX – USE SYLK A FEW MINUTES BEFORE ATTEMPTING

STEP SEVEN – ONE BD 32 HOURS FROM PEAK. BRING TIMING DOWN EACH MONTH BY ONE HOUR

STEP EIGHT – BASAL BODY TEMP – SPIKE IN TEMPERATURE SHOULD OCCUR BEFORE ATTEMPTING

STEP NINE – 12 HOURS MUST BE LEFT INSIDE THE PHASE FOR CONCEPTION TO OCCUR.

DISCLAIMER – If you are concerned over any of the supplements or lubricants we have recommended, please consult your doctor. We take no responsibility for the products chosen to use for your sway.

Our Cosmic Boy Sway Method

Knowing the effects pH has on our egg polarity and reproductive tract during the time of our surge/ovulation, whilst also aligning the ions from the Zodiacs, the chances of the gender you'll likely conceive will be male.

The timing of intercourse in relation to ovulation does matter, the pH levels in the reproductive tract (not vagina) is what sways. Negative and positive ions can alter and change our ovum's polarity, the reproductive fluids that sit around your ovum can switch between negative, neutral, and positive. Incorporating your favourable Zodiacs can help keep the eggs polarity positively charged, favouring a male sperm.

Our very own timing method was also created through years of in-house studies. From the very moment we formulated cosmic we knew our timing method had to be implemented. We knew what needed to be done, with pH being the main factor in our sway method, so we felt confident with our boy sway guidelines.

We advise having two attempts to conceive a baby boy. The reason is not only does more semen in your reproductive tract make you more alkaline, but studies also show more than one attempt yields more boys. To have more than one attempt, safely leaving enough room at the end of your phase for the sperm capacitation process to take place, the ideal time is to attempt on your **first high reading,** at the beginning of your phase. This will mean you have more time to add your second attempt safely, and your reproductive tract will be more alkaline before ovulation takes place. The cervical mucus around the time of your peak OPK will be highly alkaline EWCM {egg white cervical mucus}.

Dreaming of a bouncing baby boy? Then this is the plan for you. The abstaining rule still applies in terms of not having intercourse until you've had your peak reading, unless it's protected. This is to ensure you don't conceive in a non-favourable Zodiac. Your partner doesn't need to abstain, in fact research shows there's more male sperm when he ejaculates every other day or every four days. You must not attempt before your peak, and until you have entered the desired phase. The ideal time to peak is towards the end of the girl phase.

We must remember though that our bodies are not robots. We won't get to 1pm each month and our eggs decide it's time. Sperm waiting for the egg is key here! One month you may ovulate 26 hours after peak, and the following month it may be 34. We won't know for certainty when we ovulate, so looking at all your fertile signs is important.

Our Boy Sway Guidelines

STEP ONE – PARTNER TO RELEASE EVERY 2-4 DAYS

STEP TWO – TEST OPKS UNTIL FIRST HIGH READING PEAK IS REACHED

STEP THREE – CHECK YOUR ZODIACS

STEP FOUR – TAKE A BAKING SODA BATH EVERY DAY FOR 3 DAYS LEADING UP TO YOUR SWAY

STEP FIVE – CHECK FERTILITY SIGNS, CERVICAL POSITION & CM

STEP SIX – FIRST ATTEMPT AT HIGH READING

STEP SEVEN – SECOND ATTEMPT 12 HOURS AFTER FIRST ATTEMPT

STEP EIGHT – BASAL BODT TEMP – DO NOT ATTEMPT ON SPIKE

STEP NINE – 12 HOURS MUST BE LEFT INSIDE THE PHASE FOR CONCEPTION TO OCCUR.

DISCLAIMER – If you are concerned over any of the supplements or lubricants we have recommended, please consult your doctor. We take no responsibility for the products chosen to use for your sway.

Abstinence

Science and the success we see when your partner has abstained for between 5-10 days.

Abstinence and science shows that abstaining for seven days favours the X-bearing sperm by 2.1%. Although this doesn't sound a lot, when you calculate the extra girl swimmers in a pool of between 250 million to 40 million, 2.1% is a lot of extra Xs.

This is the one part we ask the males to do. From our extensive research in all the variables around sperm, our unpredictable biological ovulation patterns and considering the constant movement between the Moon and the Zodiacs, we are confident this is the safest method to follow without delaying fertility. Abstain seven days before ANY attempt and seven days after EVERY attempt.

Please note, although condoms can be used, we know they're not always completely safe. Our goal is for the safest possible sway for you. We want to implement abstaining seven days prior for several reasons, especially for girl swayers because we are aware of clinical studies showing that a seven-day abstaining from ejaculation period resulted in more XX chromosomes (girl sperm).

This doesn't mean this is not a safe sway for those desiring boys, because we advise more attempts take place whilst swaying boy in the male phase. And your partner can release on his own prior to attempts if needs be. But setting out a clear and precise abstaining rule we feel is very important to a successful sway.

Abstain seven days BEFORE an attempt AND seven days AFTER an attempt for the safest possible sway (all sways). Why do we need to abstain seven days after our attempt? Example: If you attempt an LFD-only sway then abstain seven days after, you can then attempt a Bio O sway as you've covered abstaining prior to that sway attempt. You've abstained, so there's no risk of crossovers fertilising the egg.

Don't forget we are talking about the potential of TWO live eggs being released in your monthly cycle. With all the variables, this is the easiest way to ensure you have a successful sway. Seven days abstaining after an attempt is also making a safer sway because you're also reducing the risk of hyper-ovulation into the wrong phase. It is why we track after ovulating to ensure our surge has ended. Other signs are the body's change in cervical mucus and the position of the cervix lowering, firming, and closing. We also have those that BBT for extra data on this. You must continue to track your LH with OPK until your numbers drop low and stay low. But for extra safety measures we advise abstaining for seven days after an attempt and you know you are covered. Keeping the rule simple and safe will leave less room for errors.

BOY SWAYERS – FREQUENT RELEASE

Abstinence is not needed for boy swayers. Instead, we recommend replenishing sperm count by releasing it every 2-4 days. This is to keep sperm healthy, motile and increase the Y sperm count. Research shows there's more male sperm when he ejaculates every other day or every four days.

How to Analyse Ovulation – Ov+8

Pinpointing ovulation down to the hour is the key to timing conception **BEFORE & AFTER** ovulation and it's not easy. Most ovulation detection methods are just designed to determine the day of ovulation, which is generally good enough to achieve (or avoid) pregnancy. For this sway, we must be ovulation experts.

Tip 1
Practice, practice, practice! Track your ovulation indicators for several practice cycles. Many times, the time of ovulation can only be determined in hindsight. Practice cycles will give you confidence that you know when ovulation is occurring and will also give you something to compare to when you're ready to make your attempt.

Tip 2
Use as many ovulation indicators as you can! No matter how regular you are, or how many cycles you practice, each cycle is different. Gather as many clues as you can to determine the real moment of ovulation. Ovulation indicators include basal body temperature (BBT), cervical mucus (CM) and ovulation prediction kit (OPK) testing.

Tip 3
Watch your CM. Your cervical mucus will usually change within hours of ovulation, changing from

EWCM to creamy or sticky. Start counting the hours when your CM has started to change.

Tip 4

Take your basal body temperature effectively. Basal body temperature is a reliable method for detecting that ovulation is truly past, so make sure to take your temperature carefully, and wait to have intercourse until you have seen your BBT shift up. However, taking your BBT once per day can only tell you that ovulation has occurred within the last 24 hours - and by then you may be too far past ovulation to conceive, because the egg only lives about 12-24 hours. You may want to try also taking a second BBT temp in the evening. It will not be as accurate as your morning "at rest" temperature, but if you take it at the same time every night after the same routine you will be able to see a pattern.

Taking your BBT in the evening in addition to the morning should help you detect ovulation within the last 12 hours. Note that your body temperature will be different in the evening - you can't compare your morning and evening BBTs to each other. You can only compare your morning temps with previous morning temps, and evening temps with previous evening temps.

Tip 5

Use OPKs as advance warning only. A positive ovulation prediction kit is a sure sign that ovulation is going to occur, but it does not give you an accurate prediction of when; it might be anywhere from 12-36 hours. When you get your first true positive OPK, begin watching your other ovulation indicators to determine exactly when ovulation is occurring.

pH

To understand why, let's first review the process of your body breaking down nutrients. Blood containing nutrients goes directly to your liver. The liver has enzymes - called cytochromes - that break down whatever they are given, including nutrients from food, medicines, and even hormones and other substances created in your body.

One cytochrome, CYP3A4, is responsible for breaking down steroid hormones, including estrogen. Estrogen is the hormone you must thank for cervical mucus. When your estrogen levels increase as you approach ovulation, your cervical mucus becomes more fertile. When estrogen levels are at their highest, your cervical mucus will be higher in alkalinity as your cervical mucus takes on that famous egg-white consistency. And after ovulation, as it begins to dry up, it will be more acidic.

pH has long been suspected of influencing the conception of a boy or a girl - it plays a crucial role in gender swaying because it's believed that an acidic pH favours X-sperms, and an alkaline pH favours Y-sperm. The argument of body pH is founded on one underlying theory: an alkaline pH in the female body favours "boy" sperm (sperm carrying the Y chromosome) while an acidic pH in the female body favours "girl" sperm (sperm carrying the X chromosome). Yin and Yang again!

pH Test Strips

Because pH plays a key role, you can check your levels of pH using disposable vaginal testing strips. This isn't always necessary, though. Some ladies like to check the levels in their vagina. It's impossible for us to test as high up into the reproductive tract, so it is important to test vaginally to give us an indication of how our pH looks during our surge.

The important thing to remember is, your vaginal CM only counts in helping the sperm on their initial journey to the egg. This can help eliminate some X or Y bearing sperm and stop them in their tracks. Based on a female's composition, higher acidity kills off the weaker boy sperm, allowing girl sperm to reach the egg, while higher alkalinity gives boys a greater chance of survival and thus greater chance to fertilise the female egg. To try to conceive a boy or a girl, you'll raise or lower the pH of the two fluids involved in conception: cervical mucus (CM), the fluid in the vagina, and semen, the fluid that carries sperm.

The pH of CM varies throughout the cycle, from very acidic to very alkaline. During the non-fertile part of your cycle, the pH of the vagina is very acidic, from 3.8 to 4.5. Approaching ovulation, the pH of CM shifts dramatically, becoming very alkaline and sperm-friendly. The varying level of pH during your cycle is very important: if CM stays too acidic, it can be a cause of infertility; if it stays too alkaline, you may be prone to yeast infections. If you are trying to conceive a girl, target a pH of 4.0-4.5 (acidic). And when trying to

The Cosmic Sway Method

conceive a boy target a pH that is between 7.5-9.0 (very alkaline).

Why Are There So Many Variables?

We believe so much in what we have created - that shows in our results! But we also believe that for most women this is their last chance at having a baby girl or a baby boy. So why not combine everything scientific to give yourself that 95% chance? When we try to fall pregnant as a natural process in life, minus swaying for a specific gender, we usually baby dance as often as possible in our fertile window. We know when we are surging, and we have a pretty good idea that ovulation has taken place too. Now add in astrology, gender selection, our unique and individual reproductive system, and don't forget sperm and capacitation.

We are trying to align all these fertility factors and join everything together, all within the correct Zodiac sign for you. Looking at all the differing variables you can see it's not a one-size-fits-all sway. We know that tracking our biological fertility pattern is something most of us have learnt whilst trying to conceive. We also know that in astrology, the Moon is your emotional center, representing the Cosmic Mother and hugely influencing our mind, body, and spirit.

Being open and awake to spirituality from a young age we learned about many different energies and auras and pattern-finding. Astrology and how it can help our everyday lives is certainly not a new concept. Tarot readers will tell you how they read male and female energies, for example, in present and/or future children.

The Cosmic Sway Method

These practices have been around for centuries. We are all able to use Mother Moon to enrich our lives.

The Biological Side

What do we need to know about the process of falling pregnant? Let's go right back to the beginning, as understanding every part of this method is hugely beneficial to you.

All these ingredients make the cake in the end: conception is the successful joining of an egg and sperm. This process can occur in the hours to days after having sexual intercourse. During sex, a male ejaculates and releases semen into the vagina (up to 250 million to be exact). Within the semen are sperm that will fight to travel out of the semen and into a woman's cervical mucus. Some sperm make it, but many will die before reaching the cervical mucus.

From here, the strongest sperm will travel to the fallopian tubes and wait for an egg to fertilise. If the two meet up, conception can occur. Even though the sperm has now fertilise an egg, there are still a few more steps that need to take place before pregnancy is successful. Conception can happen shortly after sex or several days later. Although an egg has a short life span, semen can live up to five days in the female reproductive tract. This means conception can happen in as little as a few hours and up to seven days after having sex.

After conception, the fertilised egg must move to the uterus and implant into the uterine lining or wall. This is called implantation, and it typically takes place seven to ten days after fertilisation. We will discuss natural ways to aid implantation later. We believe this is such a huge part in fertility and aiding this can make a huge difference in the time it takes you to fall pregnant.

Ovulation

Once you've come off birth control and tracked your luteinizing hormone for three consecutive months to allow you to pinpoint ovulation more precisely, you will be ready to start. We are going to advise you on the various ways to monitor and understand your monthly cycle.

The length of the menstrual cycle varies from woman to woman, but the average is to have a period every 28 days. Regular cycles that are longer or shorter than this, from 21 to 40 days, are normal. The menstrual cycle is the time from the first day of a woman's period to the day before her next period.

To understand the menstrual cycle, it helps to know about the reproductive organs inside a woman's body. These are: two ovaries - where eggs are stored, developed, and released into the womb (uterus) - where a fertilised egg implants and a baby develops; the fallopian tubes - two thin tubes that connect the ovaries to the womb; the cervix - the entrance to the womb from the vagina.

The menstrual cycle is controlled by hormones. In each cycle, rising levels of the hormone estrogen cause the ovary to develop and release an egg (ovulation). The womb lining also starts to thicken. In the second half of the cycle, the hormone progesterone helps the womb to prepare for implantation of a developing embryo. The egg travels down the fallopian tubes. If pregnancy doesn't occur, the egg is reabsorbed into the body. Levels of estrogen and progesterone fall, and the womb lining comes away and leaves the body as a period (the menstrual flow). The time from the release of an egg to the start of a period is around 10 to 16 days.

What happens during ovulation? Ovulation is the release of an egg from the ovaries. A woman is born with all her eggs. Once you start your periods, one egg develops and is released during each menstrual cycle. After ovulation, the egg lives for 24 hours. Pregnancy happens if a man's sperm meets and fertilises the egg. Sperm can survive in the fallopian tubes for up to seven days after sex, though they very rarely survive this long. Occasionally, more than one egg is released during ovulation. If more than one egg is fertilised it can lead to a multiple pregnancy, such as twins. We also know that twins are made from our *MOON EGG* being released around ovulation, also.

The 28-day female hormonal cycle mimics that of the Moon's 27.5-day cycle. Our monthly cycle begins on the first day of our period. This is akin to the New Moon. In the same way that the Moon has a waxing period leading up to the Full Moon, so too does our body. Some of the most widespread myths regarding menstruation gravitate around sex while on your period, with the top contender likely being that you cannot get pregnant while menstruating. However, this idea is entirely false. While it is true that, in many individuals, menstruation is the period when they are least fertile, it really depends on the length of their monthly cycles.

Peak fertility occurs during the ovulation stage, which usually kicks in approximately 12 to 16 days before the start of the next period, when the ovaries produce and release fresh ovules (eggs). And while most menstrual cycles last about 28 days, some cycles can be as short as 21 days, which also impacts when ovulation takes place. Moreover, sperm can live inside the genital tract for up to five days or, according to some sources, even seven days. Thus, having unprotected vaginal sex during your period could mean that the sperm gets to linger for just long enough to coincide with ovulation and fertilise an egg, resulting in pregnancy.

Recording LH

An LH surge for most women lasts between 1-3 days, with an upswing towards the surge and a downslope to return to normal baseline levels. The peak of the surge is shorter, but the entire 'surge process,' from start to finish, is generally between 1-2 days. To track correctly, it's crucial to understand your cycle length and usual ovulation day.

After tracking your cycle for a few months, you'll know how long it is (the number of days between the start of one period and the start of the next period). Most women ovulate smack dab in the middle of their cycle, and they can tell because of the type of cervical discharge they have - clear, 'egg white' discharge usually accompanies ovulation.

The best time to check LH is late morning through early evening. The LH surge is often released from the brain in the early morning, so if you get up early and test your first-morning urine, you could miss it. In addition, you should decrease fluid intake for two hours prior to ensure that your urine isn't too diluted.

The <u>first</u>, darkest line is your <u>positive/peak/surge</u>. Once your test lines show the darkest test that is visibly darker than the control line result (test line being darker than the control line), that is your surge. This means your follicle is getting ready for the egg to burst through. At this point you may experience stomach pains, change in CM, (slippery, egg white and watery, your cervix will be high up, too). Once the pain subsides, your cervical mucus will shift and become sparse, lotion-like creamy, your cervix will drop and be low.

Please also remember there are three stages to an LH pattern, and everyone is different. Most will get a peak test and then the test will lower quite soon after. Some may not and will show a continuous surge pattern! This is why testing is the absolute key to this method. You must get it right. After your peak/positive/surge, you may continue with high/peak readings for a few days, this is because some women's bodies keep hold of and store the LH. This can last for 72 hours. If you leave it this long and wait for a low before attempting, then you will miss your window.

Always go by the first surge, as this is the point in which your LH has reached a level for ovulation to occur. Unless you have a plateau surge. You'll need around 15/20 LH tests per cycle. Test at least twice a day more when you get a high reading. No fluids three hours prior to testing and hold your sample for that time too. BBT tracking for a safer, more accurate sway. Tracking cervical mucus and cervix position and texture is an advantage. Test morning and evening (minimum). Not first morning urine.

Now, this is the part where you come in: learning how to successfully find your peak in luteinizing hormone (aka LH) and know when your body is likely ovulating. LH is one of the hormones produced by the pituitary gland. It's secreted at exceptionally low levels throughout your menstrual cycle, once a developing egg follicle reaches a certain size, usually around the midpoint of your cycle. During ovulation, LH secretions surge to extremely elevated levels, as high as 7-8 - extremely alkaline.

This hormone surge is what triggers ovulation, about 12-48 hours later. Ovulation is the release of a mature egg from the ovary. It signals the beginning of your fertile period. After the egg is released, the empty follicle on the ovary is converted to a structure known as the corpus luteum. It then begins to secrete progesterone. An ovulation home test is used by women and its purpose is to help determine the time in your menstrual cycle when getting pregnant is most likely. The test detects a rise in luteinizing hormone (LH) in the urine. A rise in this hormone signals the ovary to release the egg.

This at-home test is often used by women to help predict when an egg release is likely. This is when pregnancy is most likely to occur. These kits can be bought at most drug stores. LH urine tests are different from at-home fertility monitors. Fertility monitors are digital handheld devices. They predict ovulation based on electrolyte levels in saliva, LH levels in urine, or your basal body temperature. These devices can store ovulation information for several menstrual cycles.

The specific time of month that you start testing depends on the length of your menstrual cycle. For example, if your normal cycle is 28 days, you'll need to begin testing on Day 11 (that is, the 11th day after you started your period.). If you have a different cycle interval than 28 days, talk to your health care provider about the timing of the test. In general, you should begin testing around seven days prior to the expected date of ovulation.

You will need to urinate on the test stick or place the stick into urine that has been collected into a sterile container. The test stick will turn a certain colour or display a positive sign if a surge is detected. A positive result means you should ovulate in the next 12 to 48 hours, however, this may not be the case for all women. The booklet that is included in the kit will tell you how to read the results. If you miss a day in testing there is a possibility you will miss your surge, so for that reason we suggest testing daily - three times a day.

For our method you must also test for three consecutive months - this way you can get an idea of your ovulation pattern. So, let's discuss a positive ovulation test, there is so much confusion around how the test should appear, and which is a positive reading. Firstly, if you download the app Premom this will tell you when you have reached your peak, you will note a low reading of LH and then a few peak readings, this shows your body is starting to surge. Only a <u>peak</u> reading means your test is positive and you will likely ovulate within 12-48 hours. Please note this can also happen 10-19 days after your cycle This will all depend on how long/short your luteal phase and cycle length is. You will always have a faint positive on your OPK - this is because you will always have LH in your system - it is the positive that you need to pinpoint when ovulation is near, which can be anywhere between 12-48 hours. This is what a positive and negative ovulation predictor test look like.

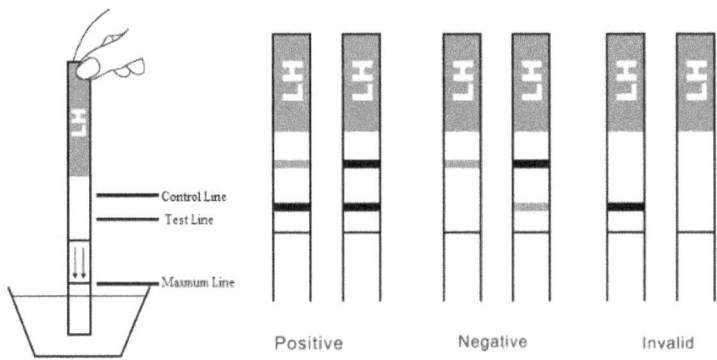

We must be mindful that there's no one rule for this, and everyone is different. There are many variables and it's what we look out for, as fertility coaches. We have clients that can ovulate multiple times in their cycles, with their biological eggs. Many have double surges too. We know what signs to look for and always advise when more, or continuous, testing needs to be done. There's so many different surge patterns and they can differ monthly for you, too. Here, we'll highlight findings from a few of our favourite studies that lead us to question what "normal" really means in the context of LH across the cycle. More specifically, we'll look at what Science has to say about these two important questions: What is a "normal" LH level on different days of the cycle? What's considered a "normal" pattern of LH around ovulation?

One large study showed that the median LH on the day before ovulation was about 44.6 mIU/mL, but that LH could be as high as 101, or as low as 6.5. Yep, some women had an LH of 6.5 the day before ovulation! Values considerably below the average lower limits and above the average upper limits might be indicative of an underlying condition that may impact ovulation. If you track your LH and discover this, it's worth bringing it up with your doctor.

Another study shows that the average LH surge was characterised by a 7.7-fold increase in LH from baseline - but LH surges ranged from 2.5-fold to 14.8-fold increases from baseline. Because the general narrative says the menstrual cycle is characterised by one quick LH surge before ovulation, you might be surprised to learn that according to some studies, *less than half* of women have LH patterns that look like that (though it is the most commonly observed out of all the noted patterns).Of studies that have characterised what patterns of LH might look like for different people, there are three recent ones that stand out as being particularly strong, and all three have converged on around the same estimates for what percent of women display which patterns:

Between 42% and 48% of cycles follow the "short surge" pattern. This is the one we're most familiar with, because this is the pattern talked about in medical textbooks and in most descriptions of the menstrual cycle.

Between 33% and 44% of cycles follow the "two surges" pattern, which - yes, you guessed it - is characterized by an initial big rise, a small drop, and then a second rise in LH.

Between 11% and 15% of cycles are characterized by the "plateau" pattern, which is when LH levels remain high after an initial surge (rather than quickly falling back down). There are other patterns as well, including multiple surges (think the two surges pattern, and then some), though they are less frequent. While some studies suggest that the pattern of LH around ovulation should look the same within an individual from cycle to cycle, others report the opposite (i.e. that LH surge characteristics differ across cycles).

Our take? If you have a short surge one cycle and a plateau next, it is perfectly normal and nothing to worry about. We cover this a little further down. Now, we know we said earlier that an LH surge indicates that ovulation is likely coming up soon, so it may be tempting to think that two LH peaks means you ovulate twice, or that a sustained high level of LH means you're ovulating for longer. Both of these are not true. For the purposes of ovulation tracking, the main thing to keep an eye out for is that initial LH surge, because it's that *initial* surge that's predictive of ovulation and peak fertility.

If you fall in the "short surge" camp, you can be confident that if you detect high LH (whatever "high" means for you), ovulation is around the corner.

But for those who fall in the "two surge" or "plateau" camp, a high LH doesn't always indicate your first LH surge - it could be indicative of a second LH surge, or of sustained high LH *after* a first surge.

We also must look out for hyperovulation; the ovaries usually release just one egg during ovulation per menstrual cycle, but sometimes, more than one egg can mature and be released by an ovary in a process called hyperovulation, which can lead to getting pregnant with multiple babies and this can result in a failed sway.

Researchers have studied ovulation and found that people may release more than one egg more often than previously thought. A 2003 Canadian study published in the *British Medical Journal* found that 40 per cent of 63 participants had the potential to produce more than one egg in any given month. Another 2003 study, published in the journal *Fertility and Sterility*, found that 68 per cent of 50 participants had two different waves of follicle development during their cycle, and 32 per cent had three.

Follicles are fluid-filled sacs that mature into eggs when there's a surge of luteinizing hormone (LH). This means that if someone has a specific hormone balance, ovulation could potentially happen multiple times, and that person could be fertile at any time of the month. The conventional belief that women ovulate once a month is wrong, say Canadian researchers who have found that women can potentially ovulate two or even three times a month. The research, published in the journal *Fertility and Sterility* (2003;80: 116-22 [PubMed] [Google Scholar]), could explain why the "rhythm" method of contraception is so unreliable and why women who take hormonal contraceptives sometimes become pregnant.

Researchers from the University of Saskatchewan did daily ultrasound scans on 63 women who apparently had normal menstrual cycles. Some were nulliparous; others had had up to three children. They found that all of the women produced at least two waves of follicular development. The existing theory held that at the beginning of each menstrual cycle, 15 to 20 follicles begin to grow in the ovaries and that one of them develops into a mature egg at roughly the middle of the cycle. Current scanning techniques can detect follicles but cannot reveal the much smaller egg itself, so it is unknown whether any of the women ovulated twice. Dr

Roger Pierson, director of the reproductive biology research unit at the University of Saskatchewan, who led the study, said 40 per cent of the subjects had the clear biological potential to produce more than one egg in a single month. Moreover, they could be fertile at any time of the month. "This really isn't the result we expected, and if it's confirmed we'll have to rewrite the textbooks," he said. "It explains why natural family planning often doesn't work, why hormonal contraception sometimes fails, and why we see fraternal twins with different conception dates."

The findings open the prospect of new approaches to contraception and assisted reproduction, Dr Pierson says. Women who take drugs to harvest eggs for in vitro fertilisation could potentially yield many more oocytes in each month. The study also calls into question the rationale for including a week of placebo pills in a monthly cycle of oral contraceptives. Professor Robert Winston, head of the department of reproductive medicine at the Hammersmith Hospital in London, said the findings were "logical and not altogether surprising."

False Surges

For most women, ovulation works as expected: follicles in your ovaries mature, the dominant one releases a single egg. During your menstrual cycle, there may be multiple waves of follicular growth, and while ovulation only happens once, the final LH surge can cause you to ovulate two (or more) eggs at the same time.

Whether through the ovaries releasing more than one egg within the same cycle (hyperovulation) or through multiple ovulations, it is technically possible to ovulate twice. While a singular rise in LH levels is most common, your egg delivery system may develop in waves, rather than once right before ovulation.

According to studies, there are three types of gradual onset LH surges (2-6 days): Confusing to track and interpret, multiple peaks in your LH surge shows several ups and downs within a cycle. There may be more than one significant rise in LH, followed by a decrease, and then a rise again. Unless you are testing and tracking your cycle, it can be difficult to recognize the right peak to know when you are fertile.

Tracking makes it easier to know exactly when ovulation has occurred, especially if you have irregular LH surges. Traditionally, it has been thought that ovulation only takes place once in every cycle. A wave of 15 to 20 egg-carrying cells, called follicles, grow before ovulation. One follicle will become dominant, and the others die off. Right before ovulation, your follicle swells up until it releases your maturing egg.

If you have multiple peaks, it may be that more than one dominant follicle is produced during a wave, or that dual conception arises because of two waves in a single cycle that release eggs. To achieve pregnancy, a follicle in the ovary ruptures and releases an egg. Regarding cases of multiple follicular stimulations, your body releases the follicle, but the follicle doesn't rupture. In this case, the egg is not released, and you are unable to get pregnant. Fortunately, your body realises that this has happened and releases a second follicle a few days later.

That's why even after one peak you can continue to see hormonal and symptom indicators of ovulation. If you're experiencing this, you should always play it safe and continue to Baby Dance before the first peak, onset, and after the second peak, as you can conceive after ovulation has taken place (i.e. conception will not result from the first follicle that was released).

Cosmic Peak

This is the term we use to identify your true peak for our girl sway method. When ladies start tracking ovulation using OPKs many ladies across most sway pages will go by their first high reading (assuming this is peak). Now, this isn't always incorrect, but we do see many that are wrong. The app you use to input your test stick data can sometimes call the wrong peak. It could be much later than it was, meaning you attempt too soon.

Sperm can also trigger LH, meaning you may attempt too early. This then brings on a stronger surge, showing a much darker test result. You could get your peak result on a morning, and from that point, ovulation occurs 12-48 hours after the LH surge is released from the brain.

You enter your LH surge (which signals ovulation) when you get your first positive (test line is usually darker than the control line). You can still be ovulating when you see your line become lighter than the control line. That doesn't mean ovulation has ended, according to all the research we have done. The LH can linger for some time or drop off almost instantly.

There's no right or wrong and everyone is very individual. We also know that reading OPKs like this is much more accurate for Ov+8. However, as previously stated for boy swayers, they can attempt from their first high reading, as sperm will likely trigger the rupture of the follicle a little sooner.

Tips and Tricks on How to Follow Your Most Fertile Signs

The following ovulation indicators help to determine the day of ovulation: Luteinizing Hormone (LH) Cervical Mucus (CM) Cervical Changes (CC) Basal Body Temperature (BBT).

LH: Ovulation tests (also known as Ovulation Predictor Kits or OPKs) are designed to detect this rise or "surge" in LH in your body. If you have never used an ovulation test kit before, here's what you can expect:

Taking the test: How you take your ovulation test will vary, depending on the type of test you have. Certain tests will require you to pee in a cup and insert a paper test strip directly into your urine, and other tests will be more like a traditional pregnancy test where you pee directly onto the test stick. Either way, try to avoid drinking too many fluids at least two hours before taking your test to ensure your urine is as concentrated as possible. This helps to improve the accuracy of your test.

Understanding your results: How your results are displayed can also vary depending on the type of test that you have. Traditional test strips will typically display two lines: one control line and one test line. A dark test line indicates that the test is "positive," and that LH is surging, whereas a lighter line indicates that the LH surge over the baseline has yet to occur. If you are using a digital test, it may display a smiley face when it detects high levels of LH.

Due to the variations in how each test works, always make sure to read the instructions thoroughly ahead of time. Try to test daily, at the same time of day. This should allow plenty of time for you and your partner to accurately time ovulation and plan for intercourse. To be able to anticipate ovulation, every woman must track their surge, peak, and ovulation as closely as possible. You can chart your CM and BBT, alongside your cervix, but for this method your LH OPK tracking is most important.

Cervical Mucus

Cervical mucus also tells us when you are highly fertile (this secretion starts in your reproductive tract - highly alkaline) and when your egg is released your CM becomes "infertile" (acidic). Don't be alarmed by the infertile CM term, you can still get pregnant when your CM is sparse, creamy, thin and lotion-like. This is the perfect CM for our girl sway.

Cervical mucus has a biological purpose. Without the presence of it, sperm would die very quickly in the vagina. Cervical mucus neutralises the pH level of the vagina, nourishes, and feeds sperm, and allows it to make the journey to the egg. Certain types of cervical mucus also filter out bad sperm, only allowing the "right" sperm to reach the egg. How cool is that?!

Cervical mucus is a hydrogel secreted by your cervical crypts. Your cervix is the entrance to your uterus, and it responds to hormonal changes throughout your cycle. Prior to ovulation, an egg is being recruited to mature while estrogen slowly builds, triggering the creation of estrogenic cervical mucus. At ovulation, estrogen is at its peak. Following ovulation is when the hormone progesterone takes over, until your next cycle, when the process starts all over again.

To start off you will need a notepad to keep track and make notes on your cervical mucus each month. Cervical mucus plays a huge part in swaying and helps you understand your cycle. Cervical mucus is great to pinpoint and determine ovulation, a few women will get around five days of egg white stretchy cervical mucus and some women get just one or two days. Therefore, it is extremely important to take note.

Once ovulation has taken place and the egg is released, your cervical mucus will start to look creamy - this is when your pH is at its lowest and female sperm thrive in a creamy acidic environment. This is the best environment to conceive a girl.

Types of Cervical Fluids

DRY
If you have no cervical fluid present at all, record your cervical fluid as "dry". You can expect to see dry days both before ovulation, after your period and after ovulation. Record "dry" if you are not able to gather or see any cervical fluid, even if your vagina feels slightly moist inside.

STICKY
Record your cervical fluid as "sticky" if it is glue-like, gummy, stiff or crumbly and if it breaks easily or is not easily stretched. It will probably be yellowish or white but could also be cloudy/clear. You may or may not see some sticky cervical fluid before and after ovulation.

CREAMY
Record your cervical fluid as "creamy" if it is like hand lotion. It could be white, yellow, cloudy, or clear. It may stretch slightly, but not very much and break easily. (Perfect for girl swayers).

WATERY
Enter "watery" if your cervical fluid is clear and most resembles water. It may be quite stretchy. This cervical fluid is considered fertile, and this may indicate your fertile window is close.

EGG WHITE
This is your most fertile cervical fluid. Record "egg white" if your cervical fluid looks at all like raw egg

white, is stretchy and clear, or clear tinged with white, or even clear tinged with pink. It resembles semen (and has a lot of the same physical properties to allow the sperm to travel and be nourished). You should be able to stretch it between your thumb and index finger. (Perfect for boy swayers).

Cervical Position

The position and texture of your cervix will change during your cycle. Wash your hands thoroughly before checking your cervix, you can easily cause an infection if you do not. During menstrual bleeding you will notice your cervix is low and hard and slightly open, it feels like the tip of your nose. When your period stops your cervix remains low and hard and the opening to the uterus remains closed.

Approaching ovulation, your cervix rises to the top of the vagina and becomes softer and moist. At ovulation, the cervix feels more like your lips than your nose and the uterine is open to allow sperm to enter. Sometimes the cervix seems to disappear – which just means it has become so soft that it blends in with the vagina walls and rises so high that the finger cannot touch it.

When ovulation is ending, your mucus will turn creamy, your cervix will also drop lower and become firmer - this is your optimal chance for a girl. And when it is open and soft is your optimal chance for a boy. In Claire's experience, she checked at around 4pm her cervix was remarkably high up – she could barely touch it. By 8.30pm her cervix was extremely low, and her CM was light and creamy (egg released in that 4.5-hour window) - that's when they attempted. Exactly 36 hours after her OPK.

That is the timing and strategy we are using with the biological side of our girl sway. Checking your cervix position whilst swaying. So, this is a really good tool to use during swaying! When the cervix is low and closed, ovulation has occurred. When the cervix is high and open ovulation hasn't occurred yet. Always make sure you wash your hands before checking.

BBT
(Basal Body Temperature)

Basal Body Temperature is the lowest body temperature attained during rest. It is usually estimated by a temperature measurement immediately after awakening and before any physical activity has been undertaken. This will lead to a somewhat higher value than the true BBT.

What Is BBT?
The Basal Body Temperature method is a technique used in family planning. Basal temperature is the temperature of your body when you are completely at rest. After a woman ovulates (releases an egg from the ovary), her body temperature rises slightly. While tracking the Basal Body Temperature during multiple menstrual cycles cannot actually predict when you are going to ovulate, it can help to establish a pattern. You will then be able to understand when you are likely to ovulate. Detecting ovulation can help you identify the days you are most likely to become pregnant. With this information, you can tell the best days to have sex if you want to become pregnant. It also helps you know which days you should avoid sex or use another birth control method to avoid becoming pregnant.

Why Is BBT Used?
People use this method to determine a woman's most fertile days of the month. Some women who want to get pregnant measure Basal Body Temperature to identify

the best days of the month to have sex. Women trying to avoid pregnancy may use it to know which days they should avoid having sex. Some women choose the Basal Body Temperature method because they do not want to take medications or hormones for birth control. In some cases, people use the method for religious reasons. In any case, it might take a while to get used to tracking and recording temperatures and to being aware of the changes in your body. Other signs that indicate where you are in your cycle include breast tenderness, pains near an ovary, and the state of your cervical mucus. Many women keep track of the day that their periods start and when they end.

How To Use BBT
- Make sure you have a thermometer that measures temperatures to at least one-tenth of a degree. This could be a regular digital thermometer or a special Basal Body Temperature thermometer.

- Take your basal temperature at the same time every day. The best time to take this temperature is immediately after waking up. Your body usually reaches its basal temperature when you are asleep.

- Measure the temperature from the same place every day. The basal body temperature can be taken in the mouth, vagina, or rectum.

- Record the temperature each day. Use a graph, list, or fertility-tracking app that allows you to compare each day's temperature.

- Identify a temperature increase. Basal Body Temperature typically rises less than ½ of a degree

Fahrenheit after ovulation. It may take a few cycles to determine when this rise occurs each month.

- <u>Consider the fertile period</u>. You are most likely to get pregnant during the period spanning two days before and three days after ovulation. If you are hoping to become pregnant, have sex during this time. If you want to avoid pregnancy, do not have unprotected sex until the fourth day after ovulation.

Girl Swayers
For girl swayers you want to start your attempt upon seeing your spike in temperature. This usually tells us ovulation has happened. A dip in temperature does not mean ovulation has occurred yet - this is important to note.

Boy Swayers
For boy swayers it's important to remember that you must not attempt once your BBT has spiked. This will bring you into girl territory and likely result in a failed sway.

Sperm

You may or may not know that the average semen lives for about 60 to - exceptionally - 72 hours. Nobody can predict exactly how long it takes the semen to travel up the birth canal to inseminate the egg. Though we have seen five and six-day cut-offs happen.

A man may ejaculate 40 million to 150 million sperm, which start swimming upstream toward the fallopian tubes on their mission to fertilise an egg. Fast-swimming sperm can reach the egg in a half an hour, while others may take days. Freshly-ejaculated sperm are unable or poorly able to fertilise. Rather, they must first undergo a series of changes known collectively as capacitation.

Capacitation is associated with removal of adherent seminal plasma proteins; reorganisation of plasma membrane lipids and proteins. It also seems to involve an influx of extracellular calcium, increase in cyclic AMP, and decrease in intracellular pH. The molecular details of capacitation appear to vary somewhat among species. Capacitation occurs while sperm reside in the female reproductive tract for a period, as they normally do during gamete transport.

The length of time required varies with species, but usually requires several hours. Sperm that have undergone capacitation are said to become hyperactivated, and among other things, display hyperactivated motility. Most importantly however, capacitation appears to destabilise the sperm's membrane to prepare it for the acrosome reaction.

Only one sperm will succeed in penetrating the egg's outer membrane. After the sperm penetrates the egg, the egg immediately undergoes a chemical reaction that prevents other sperm from penetrating. Chromosomes carried by the sperm and the egg then come together, and the egg is officially fertilised. We must use the information we have to time everything as precisely as we can, adding in all variables and increasing the chances of a successful sway.

Chemo-attractants

That's correct! The egg indeed plays a crucial role in determining your baby's sex, as it all begins with the egg itself. The egg selects sperm based on several factors, including your Zodiac compatibility, egg polarity, and pH levels.

Through a chemical process, the egg can attract the sperm it wants to allow in. Human eggs produce substances known as chemo-attractants, which help guide healthy sperm toward an unfertilised egg. For fertilisation to occur, a sperm must first merge with the plasma membrane and then penetrate the female egg cell. Consequently, sperm undergo a process called the acrosome reaction, which takes place in the acrosome as it nears the egg.

Follicular fluid surrounds the egg, sperm will then begin to alter their swimming behaviour to orient towards and accumulate in the follicular fluid, based on those chemo-attractants.

Researchers found that our eggs do not always attract the sperm from their partner compared to sperm from another male. Our eggs, on the other hand, can benefit by picking high quality or genetically compatible sperm. On average, a study found, when follicular fluid was being "more attractive" in its chemical signals, about 18% more sperm swam for their goal. And that could be "pretty important", said Professor John Fitzpatrick. There is ample evidence to show that as millions of human sperm cells swim towards a waiting ovum or egg, only one gets to fertilise it. Now, a new study shows that even though the fastest and most capable sperms reach the ovum first, it is the egg that has the final say on which sperm fertilises it.

Chemo-attractants – They Do Not Determine Your Baby's Gender

This is a new hypothesis circulating the sway forums and one we couldn't wait to debunk. Indeed, the scientists themselves make it very clear. The idea of chemo-attractants is to help the *healthy* sperm find the egg.

As we know most of us have two fallopian tubes, we release one egg, and the sperm must pick the correct tube to swim through. Chemo-attractants will send signals to the sperm to let them know where they are. Basically, shouting at the egg, I'm here, hello!! These signals really come into play when they are around 2 cm from the egg. They have nothing to do with gender selection.

Other sway pages will try and convince you that if ovulating under a male or female Zodiac, the chemo-attractant will send signals to the X or Y bearing sperm to fertilise it. (Depending on the sex you are swaying of course). We have hundreds of data to prove otherwise. In fact, most of our girl swayers ovulated in a male Zodiac and you've guessed it, they're having girls! We also have data on male babies conceived from ovulating inside a female Zodiac! When we checked their sway data, their BBT confirmed ovulation inside a female Zodiac.

The Cosmic Sway App

We understand how time-consuming it is, not to mention confusing, finding and reading the Moon phase charts online. We listened to your feedback and created our bestselling Cosmic Sway app, available via the app store and android Play store. The app will give you the days when you're in a female or male sign; colour-coded and depending on your sway preference, the days will be pink or blue. It's a fantastic tool to have on hand, it even gives you your start times and end times, so you can sway safely.

The Cosmic Sway Client Page

We have a wonderful client page for those wanting to sway the Cosmic way! We understand there are so many different methods available, and it can be extremely confusing choosing the right one. We always say to use your gut instinct when there's an important decision to be made. When something feels right, go for it. And when something feels wrong, keep looking. But we can guarantee you this: you will not find a harder working team than us. Our passion for gender swaying shows in our work ethic. Both our dreams came true with our method, and we hope to one day help you with yours.

Supplements

When we are planning on having a baby it's only natural that your thoughts turn to the idea of a little physical tune-up. Priming the body to raise it to its fertile best is a good start to making the healthiest possible baby.

There are things you and your partner can do to increase your fertility so you conceive as soon as possible. Taking natural supplements is one way both partners can prepare themselves for baby mode. First and foremost, being healthy prior to conception for both parents goes without saying. Being in the right frame of mind and in good physical health will help towards the biological side of bringing new life into this world.

The Western World seems to be catching up with the wisdom of the East in terms of natural ways to deal with a wide variety of health and wellness issues. We are rising to take control of our health and fertility naturally more than ever before. Headway in nutrition, fertility, and infertility therapy is being made daily. Drinking tea has always been associated with a healthy lifestyle and modern medicine is taking notice of the positive effects of herbal teas on reproductive health. Some of the benefits ascribed to fertility teas and herbal extracts for fertility include regulating ovulation, balancing female hormones, and nurturing the reproductive tissues.

Women the world over have known these secrets for centuries. Clinical research is now finally validating the benefits of herbs, such as Vitex (Chaste Berry) and green tea. It's also a good idea during pregnancy to take a prenatal vitamin to help cover any nutritional gaps in the mother's diet.

Prenatal vitamins contain many vitamins and minerals. Their folic acid, iron, iodine, and calcium are especially important. Folic acid helps prevent neural tube birth defects, which affect the brain and spinal cord. Prenatal vitamins are critical in supporting your baby's growth and development and your own body's changes.

However, some prenatal vitamins can cause side effects, such as nausea and constipation. You should always consult your obstetrician/gynecologist before taking prenatal vitamins. They can suggest the best prenatal vitamins with the right dosage limits based on your nutritional needs. We know we must take them before bed. It's best to start three months prior to trying to conceive.

You may be wondering why you should start supplements three months before conceiving. It takes 90 days for your eggs to develop, beginning from the time they are pulled from the waiting pool to ovulate. Prenatal vitamins are essential to pull eggs and ensure healthy development. You are aiding those eggs that will be the ones ready when you attempt this method.

Some ladies like to add extra supplements not covered in prenatal. Or they choose to just add these supplements over a combined pill. We will cover what those are and what we recommend. Don't forget the men. Of course, they are just as important when we come to making babies. After all, they have the one ingredient that makes all of this happen. Again, they can take a prenatal or fertility supplement they may wish to choose separately. Most brands are pretty much the same in terms of what they contain, the choice is down to you. And the dose will be on the packaging - it can vary, so we advise choosing one that agrees with you and follows the guidelines from the manufacturer.

Let's look at egg health first. There are two supplements we recommend in this section. Both are remarkably similar. However, girl swayers tend to avoid Coq10 as it can raise estrogen levels. Some sway myths can't be shaken, and we respect that if you'd rather choose the other, Myoinositol, that's perfectly fine. Being happy and comfortable in your pregnancy journey goes a long way.

Folate

This is the natural form of Vitamin B9, water-soluble and naturally found in many foods. Folate is also needed to produce healthy red blood cells and is critical during periods of rapid growth, such as during pregnancy and foetal development. Folate is a B vitamin which is found in some food. The man-made form is called Folic Acid and is in supplement form.

Why take Folic Acid in pregnancy? Folic Acid is a vitamin that helps your baby's neural tube grow. The neural tube is part of the baby's nervous system. Take 400 micrograms of Folic Acid every day – from before you're pregnant until you're 12 weeks pregnant. It is also recommended that you take a daily Vitamin D supplement. Do not take cod liver oil or any supplements containing Vitamin A (retinol) when you're pregnant. Too much Vitamin A could harm your baby.

Always check the label. It's important to take a 400 micrograms Folic Acid tablet every day before you're pregnant and until you're 12 weeks pregnant. If you did not take Folic Acid before you conceived, you should start as soon as you find out you're pregnant.

Try to eat green leafy vegetables which contain folate (the natural form of Folic Acid) and breakfast cereals and fat spreads with Folic Acid added to them. It's difficult to get the amount of folate recommended for a healthy pregnancy from food alone, which is why it's important to take a Folic Acid supplement. You need 10 micrograms of Vitamin D each day and should consider taking a supplement containing this amount between

September and March. Vitamin D regulates the amount of calcium and phosphate in the body, which are needed to keep bones, teeth, and muscles healthy.

NAC

N-acetyl cysteine is a supplement that simulates an amino acid called cysteine. Taking this supplement may help you get pregnant and prevent a miscarriage under certain circumstances. N-acetyl cysteine is usually safe for pregnant women to take but do ask your doctor if you are pregnant or trying to get pregnant before taking this supplement.

When you are trying to get pregnant, the most important part of your menstrual cycle is ovulation. While women stress over tracking their ovulation, NAC can ease some of that stress, as it has proven to significantly increase ovulation rates. One study found that those who took a NAC supplement during their cycle saw 52% improvement in ovulation. Pregnancy could be associated with a state of oxidative stress that could initiate and propagate a cascade of changes that may lead to pregnancy wastage. This process of oxidative stress may be suppressed by the antioxidant effect of N-acetyl cysteine (NAC).

The current study aimed to evaluate the effect of NAC therapy in patients diagnosed with unexplained recurrent pregnancy loss (RPL). The study was a prospective controlled study performed in the Women's Health Centre, Assiut University, Egypt. A group of 80 patients with history of recurrent unexplained pregnancy loss were treated with NAC 0.6g + folic acid 500 microg/day and compared with an aged-matched group of 86 patients treated with Folic Acid 500 microg/day alone.

NAC + Folic Acid compared with Folic Acid alone caused a significantly increased rate of continuation of a living pregnancy up to and beyond 20 weeks [P < 0.002, relative risk (RR) 2.9, 95% confidence interval (CI) 1.5-5.6]. NAC + Folic Acid was associated with a significant increase in the take-home baby rate as compared with Folic Acid alone (P < 0.047, RR 1.98, 95% CI 1.3-4.0). In conclusion, NAC is a well-tolerated drug that could be a potentially effective treatment in patients with unexplained RPL. Dosage between 600-1,800 milligrams of NAC daily (follow instructions on the bottle).

SUMMARY
Increases Ovulation Rates

When you are trying to get pregnant, the most important part of your menstrual cycle is ovulation. While women stress over tracking their ovulation, NAC can ease some of that stress, as it has proven to significantly increase ovulation rates. One study found that those who took a NAC supplement during their cycle saw 52% improvement in ovulation. This is compared to a previous cycle when the women took clomiphene citrate, another supplement that aims to improve fertility, where ovulation rates improved by a mere 18%.

Improves Egg Quality

NAC has also been shown to improve egg quality. This is particularly important if you are going through IVF treatments or are trying to get pregnant when you are older than 35. In a study of women suffering from PCOS, the group who received a NAC supplement saw a decrease in the amount of abnormal ovarian cells and the most significant increase in embryo quality when compared to other groups. NAC can improve the quality of your eggs and their chances of fertilisation.

Decreases Chances of Miscarriage
NAC is also proven to increase pregnancy rates in those women who experience recurrent pregnancy loss. In one study, 80 women were given a Folic Acid supplement with NAC while another 86 women were given a supplement that solely had Folic Acid. All the women in the study had a history of recurrent pregnancy loss. Those taking the supplement with NAC saw increases in the length of living pregnancy, most over 20 weeks.

Myo-Inositol

For anyone who struggles with PCOS (polycystic ovarian syndrome) or isn't ovulating regularly, studies have found taking myo-inositol may help regulate your cycles and get you pregnant faster. Myo-inositol improves insulin sensitivity and may be beneficial to add if you are experiencing delayed fertility. Cells need inositol to regulate various functions mediated by hormones and it is a vital component in the development and maturation of eggs. Although inositol occurs naturally in cereals, fruits and nuts, many women with PCOS suffer from an inositol deficiency.

Supplementing with myo-inositol can therefore assist in maintaining levels of this important nutrient. Each dose is designed to support women with PCOS or those who want to support their egg quality for preconception. Inositol is active in cell-to-cell communication, transmitting nerve impulses. Cells need inositol to regulate various functions mediated by hormones and it is a vital component in the development and maturation of eggs. Although inositol occurs naturally in cereals, fruits and nuts, many women with PCOS suffer from an inositol deficiency.

Supporting sperm health in men: Myo-Inositol supports energy production in sperm cells and sperm motility – the forward motion to get to the egg. Myo-Inositol is believed to support the function of the mitochondria within the sperm, which gives sperm energy and improves motility.

Please take the dose as stated on the bottle.

CoQ10

This is to improve your egg quality so is great for older ladies and said to increase fertilisation rates. You need to take a minimum of 600mg per day. We used to take three tablets a day. So 900mg total per day (each tablet is 300mg each). It's great for ladies over the age of 35 and said to increase fertilisation rates.

CoQ10 plays a critical role in energy production within the cells, yet the natural presence of CoQ10 in the body decreases after age 20. Research shows CoQ10 supplementation has a positive impact on pregnancy success, especially in women over the age of 35. CoQ10 is a source of energy for the eggs, supporting both egg maturation and embryo quality.

The energy contained within the egg supports embryo growth for the first 7-10 days of life, from the moment of fertilisation through to implantation. This energy drives embryo development, including the normal replication of chromosomes that results in a healthy baby. The research on CoQ10 and fertility suggests supplementation leads to more successful pregnancies.

BENEFITS OF COQ10
Promotes healthy eggs. Improves embryo quality. Prevents chromosomal defects. Increases successful pregnancies. Extra CoQ10 is particularly helpful in situations where the quality of the eggs may already be compromised, including: diminished ovarian reserve, PCOS (polycystic ovarian syndrome), endometriosis, painful periods.

While our bodies do make CoQ10, natural production decreases with age. CoQ10 is available in food from sources like fatty fish, organ meats and whole grains. However, the amount of CoQ10 reasonably sourced from food is often insufficient to maintain optimal levels in the body for fertility. Supplements can provide the levels needed to promote fertility and a healthy pregnancy.

Ginger

Due to its anti-inflammatory properties, ginger is beneficial for women struggling with fertility issues. Inflammation can negatively impact the female reproductive system because it reduces blood circulation, which is necessary for ovulation, menstruation and fertilisation. Ginger has been shown to be useful for promoting both male and female fertility.

Antioxidant
Studies show that ginger contains incredible antioxidants that protect cells from oxidative stress and damage. Oxidative stress can affect egg cells leading to ovulatory infertility. The antioxidant effects of ginger can combat this and help promote fertility.

Anti-inflammatory
Ginger is well-known for its powerful anti-inflammatory properties because of its main active ingredient, gingerol. Infertility related reproductive conditions like PCOS, or endometriosis, are linked to and further aggravated by too much inflammation in the body.

Promotes blood circulation
In traditional Chinese and Ayurvedic medicine, ginger is a warming herb. This means, when consumed it warms up the body because it boosts blood flow in the body. By circulating and delivering nutrient-rich blood to your reproductive system, it enhances healthy reproductive function and clears away toxins as well.

Ginger is available fresh or dried in powdered form/capsules/as a tea. You may consume ginger in any form that's available to you. Here are easy ways to consume ginger for fertility:

As a tea: this is by far the most wonderful way of consuming ginger. Simply steep an inch of freshly shaved ginger into a cup of boiling water for five minutes. Then strain the tea, add in 1tsp of organic honey and sip away! You can replace your morning caffeine with this simple ginger tea.

Capsules: ginger capsules are available to take as a supplement. It helps with inflammation, pain, and digestive support.

Powder form: ground ginger or dry ginger powder can be used to make tea by steeping about ¼ to ½ tsp in a cup of boiling water for five minutes. Sweeten with honey and enjoy!

In Smoothies: add about ½ to 1 inch of freshly peeled ginger into your smoothies when blending.

In cooking: so many recipes use fresh or dried ginger to season so feel free to add ginger into your cooking! Ginger + garlic is one of the best combos when it comes to seasoning practically any savoury dish.

Vitamin D

Vitamin D3 (cholecalciferol) is the main form of Vitamin D; it is in the skin, and it can be found in some food and nutritional supplements. Prescription Vitamin D is Vitamin D2 (ergocalciferol). In general, research shows that we metabolise Vitamin D3 more efficiently than Vitamin D2.

Vitamin D has been linked to a variety of health benefits. For women trying to conceive, it appears to be linked to better fertility, as well as a healthy pregnancy. Several studies have found that Vitamin D blood levels of 30 ng/mL or higher are associated with higher pregnancy rates. Two studies found that among populations of mostly Caucasian and non-Hispanic white women, those with a normal Vitamin D level were four times more likely to get pregnant through IVF compared to those who had a low Vitamin D level.

Another study found that donor egg recipients with a normal Vitamin D level had higher pregnancy rates than those with a low Vitamin D level. Most fertility supplements only contain about 400 IU of Vitamin D. While this may be enough for some women, it may not be enough for others to ensure their Vitamin D levels are in a healthy range. Some research indicates that taking 2000-4000 IU of Vitamin D daily is not only safe, but is recommended for women, especially those who are pregnant.

Vitamin E – 400mg

This strengthens the outer shell of the egg and helps with implantation. However, Vitamin E can increase EWCM production for some people. Using Vitamin E for fertility will enhance blood flow in parts of the body essential for alleviating this issue when taken in quantities of around 400mg per day. This will result in increased thickness and is part of the reason why Vitamin E works well as a fertility vitamin.

Vitamin E was first discovered in 1922 as a substance necessary for reproduction. Following this discovery, Vitamin E was extensively studied, and it has become widely known as a powerful lipid-soluble antioxidant.

There has been increasing interest in the role of Vitamin E as an antioxidant, as it has been discovered to lower body cholesterol levels and act as an anticancer agent. Numerous studies have reported that Vitamin E exhibits anti-proliferative, anti-survival, pro-apoptotic, and anti-angiogenic effects in cancer, as well as anti-inflammatory activities.

There are various reports on the benefits of Vitamin E on health in general. However, despite it being initially discovered as a vitamin necessary for reproduction, to date, studies relating to its effects in this area are lacking.

*Please note this can lean towards a boy sway - only add this if you're experiencing delayed fertility.

Vitamin B12 – 150 mcg

This makes folic acid work better (B6 also lengthens luteal phase. If you take B6 and get a BFP don't stop suddenly, rather decrease it slowly). Vitamin B12 is a key vitamin to increase your fertility. Vitamin B12 enhances the occurrence of ovulation, being particularly helpful to women not ovulating at all, making it harder to try to conceive.

If you did not already know, Vitamin B12 is a vital component for methylation and Vitamin B12 deficiency can lead to high homocysteine levels. Studies show that a Vitamin B12 deficiency creates an imbalance in one carbon metabolism - a process involving folate, MTHFR, and homocysteine - that decreases female fertility and compromises the ability for fertilised embryos to implant themselves in the uterus. High homocysteine levels are associated with a variety of fertility and health problems.

Increased Risk of Miscarriage
Miscarriage is common among people who are deficient in Vitamin B12, due to associated high homocysteine levels and methylation problems. Elevated homocysteine levels drastically increase the risk of developing blood clots during pregnancy, and in many cases, clots that occur during pregnancy are what leads to miscarriage.

Irregular Ovulation
A regular ovulatory cycle is important for fertility because it gives you a greater chance at accurately

predicting when you are most fertile. If Vitamin B12 deficiencies are chronic, women seeking to become pregnant will also experience inconsistent ovulatory cycles, changes to the development of the ovum, and experience chronic implantation issues.

Increased Risk of Neural Tube Defects
Neural tube defects are more prevalent in women with Vitamin B12 deficiencies due to how closely Vitamin B12 relates to the folate cycle. Vitamin B12 and the active form of folate is needed to convert homocysteine to methionine. Without enough Vitamin B12, homocysteine begins to rise, leading to previously mentioned fertility problems, but also methylation issues arise due to low methionine levels. A growing foetus requires a lot of methylation to coordinate its growth effectively, especially its nervous system, and without adequate folate and Vitamin B12 levels there is an increased risk of developing neural tube defects.

Zinc – 50mg

This repairs any of the eggs that may have been damaged and helps with implantation. Zinc is the substance that is known to have the greatest influence on fertility and is effective both in male and female patients that have fertility issues. Zinc is a basic element that makes up genetic material, and if there is a deficit in the body, this will clearly affect fertility. Zinc is also required to produce healthy eggs in women.

Animal studies involving zinc and reproduction have "consistently shown a zinc requirement for oocytes" (female egg cells) for various processes like cell division, fertilisation, and embryo development. According to researchers, this is why the role of zinc is so important in measuring the quality of an ovum to improve fertility therapies in the future.

In addition, zinc can help reduce the size of fibroids, which are often responsible for fertility problems, and regulate hormone levels. There are many supplements, teas, foods we can add to boost fertility naturally and help maintain a healthy pregnancy, we have just listed our personal favourites,

There's also a huge selection that will aid male fertility, such as CoQ10 for example. Scientists believe CoQ10 functions as an antioxidant that blocks actions that can damage cells. Decreased sperm motility is one of the leading causes of male infertility, but there's a noteworthy treatment option that may make a difference. Studies have found that supplements of CoQ10 can help improve sperm movement in infertile men. According to some research, the amount of CoQ10 in the seminal fluid of men has a correlation to their sperm count and sperm motility.

Vitex

(Vitex agnus-castus) is a plant used in herbal medicine. Also known as Chaste Tree or Chaste Berry, it's often taken as a remedy for women's health problems. Vitex supplements typically contain extracts of the fruit and/or seed of the plant.

Vitex may influence hormone levels in several ways. For example, it's said to promote the release of luteinizing hormone and, in turn, increase levels of progesterone (a hormone known to play a key role in regulating the menstrual cycle). Vitex is also thought to affect levels of prolactin, which is involved in stimulating breast development and milk production in women.

A nutritional supplement containing a blend of vitex, green tea, L-arginine, vitamins (including folate), and minerals may help improve fertility in women, suggests a study published in *Clinical and Experimental Obstetrics & Gynaecology* in 2006. The study involved 93 women (ages 24 to 42) who had tried unsuccessfully to conceive for six to 36 months. Three months into the study, 26 per cent of the study members treated with the Vitex-containing supplement had become pregnant (compared to just 10 per cent of those given a placebo).

This finding indicates that nutritional supplements could provide an alternative or adjunct to conventional fertility therapies, according to the study's authors. Vitex is safe to take when trying to conceive - some studies show that Vitex in early pregnancy can decrease miscarriage but for the most part it has been inconclusive. But there are some people that take it until the end of the first trimester.

We decided to wean off Vitex at 12 weeks when the placenta takes over. Use of Vitex should be avoided for those with hormone-sensitive conditions (such as endometriosis, uterine fibroids, and cancers of the breast, ovaries, or prostate). These shouldn't take Vitex without consulting a practitioner who is knowledgeable in its use. As with anything we take, please follow the recommended guidelines on dosage and consult a health practitioner if you're nursing or on prescription medication.

Vitex is a genus of flowering plants in the sage family Lamiaceae. It has about 250 species. Common names include Chaste Tree or Chaste Berry, traditionally referring to V. agnus-castus but often applied to other species as well. For fertility, Vitex increases luteinizing hormone production while mildly inhibiting the release of follicle stimulating hormone (FSH). This indirectly boosts progesterone production and the chances of achieving and maintaining a successful pregnancy. Vitex decreases high prolactin levels, which are associated with breast pain.

Sex Selection Supplements

Something we are often asked is which supplements favour the two genders. Again, we have investigated this extensively and we do not say it is necessary to add extra supplements unless you want to. However, we do believe in the studies we have found and believe they can give a helping hand. We look at our method as a combined approach including astrology and biology to give the highest success rates.

Girl Sway Supplements
Let's start with our favourite. Calcium and Magnesium Citrate. It must be citrate. And here's why…

There is a lot of talk across the internet which has debunked calcium and magnesium for swaying girl, but we don't believe this to be true. So let's discuss calcium and magnesium citrate: these supplements were once used many moons ago to help aid natural gender selection, they have now been "debunked" by many sway forums and groups as they seem to believe that this sways boy.

Many groups and forums claim that these supplements will give your body added nutrients and minerals that will help the XY to thrive. It's somewhat true, however, some are unsure what to use so take the incorrect calcium (calcium carbonate) during their girl sway. This is an alkaline-based mineral that requires extra stomach acid for better absorption - these will sway boy due to the alkalinity in them.

Calcium citrate is an acidic-based mineral and does not need extra stomach acid for absorption, so these will sway girl. Some groups have accumulated a small number of statistics in which they believe that calcium and magnesium citrate may have potentially been the reason some sways failed. However, when looking at these statistics, it's clear that when these supplements were used and sways failed there were several other factors that contributed in these results, for example, most of the sways had cut-offs 5,4,3,2 days before ovulation (timing), some never tested pH levels and we know that intercourse around your LH surge increases pH which favours the XY, plus the diet wasn't completely girl-friendly.

We can confidently say this, as all our sways have taken calcium and magnesium citrate; they have followed our method and the failure rate is extremely low, so it goes without saying that they are not the overall factor for a failed sway. You cannot debunk science, right?

These supplements were tested for natural gender selection in a laboratory in 2011, rats were used for this experiment, and this showed an impressive result with an 82% success rate, opposed to the rats who were given no supplements, and the result showed 48.64%. Furthermore, these supplements were used for all our sway cases and showed a huge success rate. Most calcium citrates will contain Vitamin D3, a low dose of this is fine.

Calcium carbonate could be down to girl sway fails, due to the alkalinity causing the ovum polarity to switch, so these are not advised. A study performed in a clinical trial for gender swaying, showed that of those who fasted and took calcium and magnesium citrate during the month they conceived, 80% had girls as opposed to those who did not take the supplements conceived 50:50 on the gender.

By changing the intake of key minerals through supplements, the concentration of these minerals in the blood changes, which then increases the odds for conceiving a specific gender.

Calcium Citrate x 1200mg daily

Magnesium Citrate x 200mg daily

Please note this is a guideline. It is sometimes not possible to get the exact quantity so you can take a little less or a little higher of each dose. We advise not to go over 400mg of Magnesium Citrate daily.

Boy Sway Extras

Something we are often asked is which supplements favour the two genders. Again, we have investigated this extensively and we do not say it is necessary to add extra supplements unless you want to. However, we do believe in the studies we have found and believe they can give a helping hand. We look at our method as a combined approach including astrology and biology to give the highest success rates.

Boy Swaying supplements & drinks
We've mentioned pH and cervical mucus and how those sway in relation to the Moon phases and our reproductive tract and vaginal environment. You can also create a perfect boy-friendly environment in addition to lunar fertility.

Fish Oil 500mg x1 daily
These particular fatty acids can help decrease inflammation in the body and can improve blood flow. They can also increase cervical mucus. Essential fatty acids play an important role in regulating hormones, increasing the blood circulation to the uterus, increasing the quantity of the cervical mucus and so on. If your daily diet isn't rich in essential acids such as Omega 3, 6 and 9, then it's time for you to include nutritional supplements such as Evening Primrose Oil, Borage Seed Oil, and L-arginine in your diet.

Guaifenesin
One spoonful daily in your fertile window for five consecutive days. Stopping after ovulation. Guaifenesin is reputed to "thin" cervical mucus - the fluid produced by a woman's cervix during her ovulatory cycle. Cervical mucus plays an important role in human reproduction, providing a fertile, protective medium that allows sperm to move through the cervical canal, swim the expanse of the uterus, and ultimately fertilise the egg. For cervical mucus to exhibit "fertile" properties - emerging around the time a woman ovulates - the fluid must be both abundant and sufficiently thin (or viscous instead of thick and sticky). In addition, fertile-quality cervical mucus will alter the pH-balance of the vagina to make a normally acidic, sperm-hostile environment into a "sperm-friendly" setting commensurate with successful baby-making.

Add carrots to your diet
There are several foods to increase the quantity of cervical mucus, and carrots are one of them. Carrots are rich in beta-carotene, which aids in creating Vitamin A in the human body. Foods rich in Vitamin A help to not only increase the quantity of cervical mucus but also improves its quality.

Green tea
Yum, drink one cup a day starting from the first day of your period until ovulation. Why? It increases overall fertility, and you've guessed it, cervical mucus. Your green tea will help hydrate your body so that it is better prepared to produce the cervical fluid your body needs to get pregnant more easily.

Evening Primrose Oil

Evening Primrose may have a wide range of beneficial effects for fertility. Because it is rich in Omega 6 essential fatty acids, linoleic acid, and gamma linolenic acid, it is thought to be effective in reducing inflammation, relieving PMS, increasing production of cervical mucus, and improving overall uterine health.

Oil of Evening Primrose helps increase fertility by helping your body produce fertile cervical mucus and helps to regulate your ovulation menstrual cycles. The quality and quantity of your CM is important to getting pregnant. As you approach ovulation, your cervical fluids should become more abundant and of a quality that nurtures the sperm. It should become thinner, watery, and have the consistency of egg whites. This provides the best environment for sperm to be able to travel to the fallopian tubes and be nourished to survive longer while they await an egg to be released.

Oil of Evening Primrose will also help to soften the cervix which encourages the opening of the cervix to be wider. This, obviously, will help more sperm to be able to travel through to the uterus and fallopian tubes.

It is generally accepted that the dosage needed for *fertility* issues and/or PMS is 1500mg to 3000mg per day taken in one dose in the morning by mouth, not to exceed 8g in one day or 24-hour period. Higher doses may be prescribed for more severe conditions. Consult your healthcare provider of certified herbalist.

EPO is available as an oil or in capsules and should be kept in the refrigerator and out of direct sunlight to prevent the oil from becoming rancid. Generally, high-quality oil will be certified as organic by a reputable third party, packaged in light-resistant containers, refrigerated, and marked with a freshness date.

EPO should be standardised to contain 8% gamma-linolenic acid. Primrose oil should not be taken if you have bleeding problems or a blood disorder. It should not be taken with certain psychiatric medications such as those prescribed for schizophrenia. Also not for use with non-steroidal anti-inflammatory drugs (NSAIDs) like ibuprofen. Evening primrose is not considered to be safe if used in pregnancy.

Some midwives may use it to ripen the cervix during the 3rd trimester of pregnancy, to make it ready for delivery. Either evening primrose oil is rubbed on the female's cervix, or it is taken internally, or it is used as a vaginal suppository. We advise to stop taking after ovulation and start again on CD1. You are not advised to continue taking the supplement after ovulation, as evening primrose may cause contractions in your uterus, making it difficult for the egg to get implanted in the womb. During the luteal phase after ovulation, it may be suggested to take Omega-3 fish oil supplements to support your overall health. Please be aware it can also change your cycle length and some ladies do use this to delay ovulation to line up in a boy phase. Take the recommended dosage of evening primrose every day until your ovulation occurs. You must swallow the whole capsule with a glass of water.

Grapefruit juice
One glass a day to increase cervical mucus. Grapefruit contains chemicals called furanocoumarins. When they are absorbed into the blood and sent to the liver, furanocoumarins temporarily disable CYP3A4. This

means that for a short period of time, a few hours, perhaps, your body doesn't have what it needs to break down estrogen. For this reason, estrogen hangs out in your body for a bit longer than it normally would, causing estrogen levels in your body to be higher.

There are also many doctors and midwives who tell their patients to drink grapefruit juice to help along the fertilisation process. Due to the healthy vitamins and nutrients found in grapefruit juice, it can also be helpful to drink it for the Vitamin C. Natural Fertility Info shared that grapefruit juice contains a good amount of Vitamin C, which improves hormone levels and increases fertility in those with luteal phase defect, according to a study published in *Fertility and Sterility*.

According to the Federal Drug Administration (FDA), grapefruit juice can interfere with certain medications, allowing more of the drug to enter your bloodstream. This all comes back to grapefruit juice's ability to disable the CYP3A4 cytochrome, which is also responsible for metabolising and breaking down drugs in your system. The FDA explained that when grapefruit juice blocks CYP3A4 in the small intestine, it allows more of the medication to enter your blood and lets it stay there longer, resulting in too much medication in the system. So, if you are taking any medications, you should definitely talk to your doctor or pharmacist about any possible reactions or interactions grapefruit juice may cause.

For Your Partner

Vitamin D

Vitamin D and fertility for men. Maintaining a normal Vitamin D level is not only important for women trying to conceive. It can benefit the male partner as well. Studies have found a direct relationship between Vitamin D levels and an improved ability of sperm to begin a pregnancy, both during ovulation induction and timed intercourse. Please take the amount as recommended on the bottle.

Green tea

Share the joy. This cup of magic contains polyphenols, whose antioxidant activities could improve sperm parameters and fertility. The sperm production rate, sperm count and overall fertility of any male is influenced by several factors, including nutrition and lifestyle.

It's also affected by the actions of free radicals within the body.

Sperm by its nature is very susceptible to free radicals. These are highly reactive toxins in the body which cause oxidative damage to body cells and DNA. Some of these free radicals can be neutralised by the actions of antioxidants present in green tea. As a result, the tea will help improve male fertility.

Men who drink green tea should naturally experience a higher sperm count than those who avoid tea or drink it less frequently.

Zinc

Zinc is a trace mineral needed by the human body in tiny amounts to maintain good health. In addition to preventing zinc deficiency, many people take zinc supplements for a variety of reasons, including boosting the immune system and preventing heart disease. Although zinc is generally safe and well-tolerated, large doses of zinc may cause a variety of side effects, including dizziness.

Several studies proposed the importance of zinc in male fertility. Low zinc or zinc deficiency can negatively influence several factors that are directly related to male fertility, like low testosterone and decreased sperm quality. Zinc is a mineral with antioxidant properties that play a critical role in sperm development. We advise to start three months prior to trying to conceive as sperm can take approximately 90 days to develop fully.

The Office of Dietary Supplements states an adult male needs <u>11 milligrams of zinc daily</u>. Your body has no storage capacity, so you need to get the recommended amount every day through diet or supplementation.

As for men with sperm abnormalities, 25 to 50 mg of zinc have been shown to increase sperm count and boost testosterone levels.

Girl Sway Lubricants

Why use them? Most lubricants are sperm-friendly, and these can be used to help as part of your sway. A lubricant can be used to help create the right environment within the vagina before your attempt.

Let's cast our minds back to pH. We know male sperm favour the higher alkalinity environment and females thrive in an acidic environment. We also know that the reproductive tract is where it counts the most. But we also know that sperm must travel through the vagina before it hits the cervix and eventually the reproductive tract.

So why not make that short journey favourable for them? We are, after all, talking about millions of sperm and the less amount of the gender we are not swaying for, the better. We aren't talking here about douching nor are we talking about using anything that is not healthy either. But we can create the right environment for your vagina before your attempt.

Of course, like any of the things we recommend in this chapter it is down to personal choice and we don't say they're necessary to do this method. Many couples will use a lubricant during sexual intercourse, that's nothing new. We have just found the right one for you that will lean more pink or blue.

We do have to mention that, like anything, we use topically, and we must stop using something if there's any adverse side effects. We have two for those wanting a baby girl. We have used these personally and we see remarkable results when used compared to other lubricants/gels.

'RepHresh' Vaginal Gel

Many vaginal problems are caused by an imbalance in vaginal pH. An unbalanced pH can be caused by common occurrences such as your period, unprotected sex, douching or the hormonal changes you experience during pregnancy. The good news is that balanced vaginal pH is important for maintaining good vaginal health. And that's where RepHresh comes in.

RepHresh is an over-the-counter vaginal gel clinically proven to maintain healthy vaginal pH. It's colourless, odourless, and long-lasting - just one application lasts for three full days.

'Sylk' Lubricant

Sylk is an intimate, plant-based lubricant that provides relief from vaginal dryness. A water-soluble, pH friendly lubricating gel, Sylk is kind and gentle to sensitive tissues. Suitable for everyday dryness and lovemaking. Safe to use with condoms. A few drops of Sylk can aid tampon insertion. Claire used this in her successful girl sway along with hundreds of ladies across the gender sway pages, and it comes out on top. You may want to purchase ahead of time as ladies outside of the UK can have long periods to wait for stock to be replenished. It sells like hot cakes.

Sylk lubricant is recommended as part of this sway and should be the only one used. After ejaculation your partner's sperm is extremely alkaline, this lubricant will help the X-bearing sperm have a head start, the girl swimmers will thrive in the acidic lubricant whilst the

XY will not. Studies show the X sperm favours acidity, and Y sperm favours alkalinity. No other lubricants or douches should be used for this method. Other lubricants on the market have a much lower pH level - this could ultimately hinder your chances to conceive by killing the sperm off completely or causing vaginal infections. The amount you use depends on your own personal preference. You can insert it into the cervix using a syringe or a fingertip. This is to be used prior to your attempt.

Boy Sway Alkalinity

Baking Soda Bath
The alkaline nature of baking soda is said to help draw out toxins from the body. A baking soda detox bath is said to promote sweat, neutralise skin acidity, and may aid in boosting immunity and overall health. While research on the exact effects of baking soda detox baths is few and far between, anecdotal evidence suggests they might promote relaxation, detoxification, and general well-being.

It can also help raise your pH levels within your vagina. This is favourable in the sway world for boy swayers. We recommend adding ¼ cup of baking soda to a bath and soak for 15 to 20 minutes prior to your attempts. This can be done for three days leading up to your sway, also.

Delaying Ovulation
We have decided to add this as we are asked this question daily. How do I delay ovulation to line up in the girl phase? You can take a period delay pill which will move your next ovulation day. We must advise that we don't actively ask ladies to alter their monthly cycles or change their hormones to delay ovulation. However, many of our clients would like more opportunities in the girl phase and would like to change their ovulation day.

Period Delay Pill
So, this is something some ladies choose to take when they've noticed the month ahead will put their ovulation in the boy phase. We've researched this extensively and we are aware that the brand we advise on is only available on prescription in some locations. In the UK it can be bought online. You will be able to source an alternative by searching what's available in your country.

Norethisterone
Norethisterone, also known as norethindrone and sold under many brand names, is a progestin medication used in birth control pills, menopausal hormone therapy, and for the treatment of gynaecological disorders. The medication is available in both low-dose and high-dose formulations and both alone and in combination with an estrogen. It is used by mouth or, as norethisterone enanthate, by injection into muscle.

Postponement of menstruation by mouth for females of childbearing potential: take 5mg three times a day, to be started three days before expected onset (menstruation occurs 2–3 days after stopping). Norethisterone tablets are pills you can take to stop and delay your period. Norethisterone tablets need to be taken three days before you expect your period to begin and delay your period until about three days after you have taken the last tablet.

Aiding Implantation

Once we've swayed and we have landed in the Zodiac phase for the gender we desire, we want that pregnancy to take place. We all know how frustrating it can be when ovulation doesn't land in the boy or girl Zodiac, and when it does, we want that to be our month. The problem many ladies face when trying to conceive is the implantation side. It's the biggest reason for infertility. The embryo is formed, but for different reasons it can't nestle into your womb. It then dies off and we get our AF (Aunt Flow).

Usually when trying for a baby, we get a few cycles before we catch and the monthly menstruation is heavy, with clots and a fuller flow. We firmly believe this is down to the embryo not implanting as the cycles are usually very light. So, what we need to look at, when our sway has been safe and ticks all the boxes, is getting that embryo to implant. The most common reason it won't is that the lining is too tough. This can be from scar tissue if you've ever had any procedures, PCOS, endo and sometimes it can be down to diet. We want to make the lining soft and easy for the embryo to implant.

Imagine it's tough, thick, and firm, it's going to be harder for a tiny, delicate embryo to nestle in and pregnancy to take place. With the usual losses we have along the way you start to research the best way for a sticky baby.

The things we've used over the years to help have all been natural, apart from aspirin. So, we must always be careful when we add anything to our bodies. We've worked with natural remedies for many years including herbs, supplements, oils etc. And we can honestly say the results are astounding. Not just in the TTC world but we've spent many years heavily involved in holistic remedies and research. These are the top ones we would recommend for aiding implantation:

Bromelain

You can take two tablets daily starting from 2DPO until 5DPO (days past ovulation). Take the dose on your bottle. There's no right or wrong. But be mindful that some prenatals have this ingredient in so you won't need the highest dose. Pineapple is an implantation "wonder fruit". It contains the antioxidizing enzyme *bromelain*, which is a powerful anti-inflammatory. When it comes to the implantation of an embryo, having balanced hormones is not enough – the uterus needs to be prepared and receptive to the embryo. The bromelain in pineapples helps to lessen the inflammation in the uterus, making implantation more likely to be successful.

Brazil Nuts

Brazil nuts are a fantastic source of *selenium*, which is a mineral that thickens the uterine wall and promotes a healthy uterine lining – both of which aid implantation. Additionally, selenium is a natural anticoagulant that helps to increase blood flow to the uterus and ovaries. Also, it helps to prevent blood clots from forming that could cause a miscarriage.

To benefit from Brazil nuts, you should eat about two or three Brazil nuts each day from the first day of ovulation until at least ten days post ovulation. Only eat them fresh or raw. Do not roast or cook them.

Pomegranate

Fresh fruit equivalent only. Drinks in supermarkets etc won't be the right level you need. You can eat the seeds, but you'd need tonnes. We recommend a supplement for this reason (We've used the fresh concentrated juice and it's not pleasant). We advise to start this from 3DPO until 6DPO because it can cause the thinning of blood, and we want to ensure the embryo is formed prior to starting.

Pomegranate juice is a dark red nectar that helps to increase blood flow. It also has anti-inflammatory properties! This fruit combines the benefits of pineapples and Brazil nuts.

For that reason, ancient Persians considered pomegranates to be a symbol of fertility. The fruit is full of antioxidants and micronutrients necessary for implantation, such as Vitamin C, folate, and Vitamin K. The suggested "dosage" of pomegranate juice is 1 cup of 100% pomegranate juice daily throughout your menstrual cycle to get the most benefits from the super juice.

I personally take all these in supplement format: Bromelain, and pomegranate. I also drink the following teas to aid implantation, lavender, and raspberry leaf tea. Drinking plenty of water is also exceptionally good and promotes egg health.

Aspirin

So again, this is a blood thinner and an anti-inflammatory and it's why it's successful in TTC. There are tonnes of research on this as it makes your reproductive environment perfect for a sticky baby.

You only need a low dose. You may hear it referred to as "baby Aspirin" for this reason -75mg daily is sufficient. You can start this in your fertile week, some take it all cycle, or you can take it after ovulation and stop at a BFP or AF.

Water
Drinking plenty of water is always a good thing but especially when we are trying to get a pregnancy to stick. We don't want to be dehydrated.

Staying Warm
IVF clinics will advise on this. It's going to help the embryo implant as the warmer we are, the cosier the environment will be. Get some fluffy socks and keep those trotters warm. We lose so much heat through our feet, so stay snuggled.

Diet
Think of foods high in progesterone. You don't have to go overboard but add some salmon, some green leafy vegetables and avocado is great. Nuts are also brilliant as they're also packed with B vitamins. You can also drink herbal teas.

Just be mindful that you don't need to overdo this. If anything upsets your tummy, then limit it or cut it out - Green tea, red raspberry leaf tea to name a couple. Think of helping your digestive tract, so probiotic drinks. Kefir is my favourite, it's more natural. Also pumpkin and sunflower seeds.

Iron-rich foods are very important to help implantation. They boost blood supply to the uterus and help build up the lining which encourages pregnancy. Anti-inflammatory foods should be included in your entire diet to promote healthy implantation. As stated earlier, an inflamed uterus is not suitable for conception. Some anti-inflammatory foods you can choose include: olive oil, tomatoes, leafy greens like spinach, kale, and collards and seeds like almonds, walnuts, and black sesame seeds, fatty fish like salmon, fruits like strawberries, blueberries, cherries, and oranges.

In Chinese medicine, Kidney Jing is incredibly important. It is what nourishes and provides for the reproductive system. According to Zhang Jie Bin, a well-known Chinese doctor: *"There are two kidneys (kidney yin and yang), with the Gate of Vitality between them. The kidney is the organ of water and fire, the abode of yin and yang, the sea of essence, and it determines life and death."*

Bone broth, roasted bone marrow, stews, slow cooked meats help to support and replenish Kidney Jing. All nuts and seeds, Caviar, seaweeds, and algaes – including spirulina and chlorella beans, eggs, oysters, organ meats like liver, heart, and kidneys.

Progesterone
Progesterone is known as the "pregnancy hormone". Progesterone helps the fertilised egg be implanted in the uterus to establish a pregnancy and help maintain a healthy pregnancy. Women naturally produce progesterone in the ovaries, the placenta, and the adrenal glands during pregnancy. During fertility treatments such as IVF (in vitro fertilisation), progesterone is often given because the medications used in the process reduce a woman's natural production of the hormone.

Progesterone is a hormone created early in pregnancy by a cyst on the ovary called the Corpus Luteum. This cyst of the ovarian follicles continues to produce progesterone for ten weeks during pregnancy. After those initial weeks, then the placenta takes over producing progesterone. During the first trimester, progesterone levels rise exponentially, but plateau shortly after.

Progesterone is key to creating a perfect environment for the ovaries to harbour the foetus by keeping the uterus muscle relaxed and helping the immune system tolerate foreign DNA. When a woman undergoes IVF or another fertility treatment, this hormone will sometimes need to be supplemented. Women's ovarian follicles might also be poorly developed and may not secrete enough progesterone on their own. In these circumstances, progesterone will need to be supplemented as well.

Before Pregnancy
The hormone progesterone is secreted during early pregnancy and prepares the uterus for pregnancy. It causes the luteal phase to start and transforms the endometrium (uterine lining) by thickening it to receive an embryo. The embryo is the result of the female's egg when it's fertilised by the male's sperm. When pursuing pregnancy, the fertilised embryo will reach the uterus normally five days after ovulation. Then two days later, it will attach to the uterine wall. After it attaches to the uterine wall, this is when progesterone levels peak. If undergoing IVF, the client would normally go through progesterone supplementation to help encourage the fertilised embryo to attach to the uterine wall.

During Pregnancy
Progesterone helps support the foetus as it grows. When a woman is pregnant, they produce hCG (human chorionic gonadotropin hormone). This is a signal to the ovaries to continue to produce progesterone. hCG prevents the onset of her menses (the blood and matter discharged during ovulation) and enables a woman to become pregnant. Progesterone then continues to be produced, nurturing the foetus as it starts to grow. After 8-10 weeks of pregnancy, the placenta takes over progesterone production and increases production until the baby is born.

Benefits
Estrogen, the primary female sex hormone, stimulates the growth of tissue inside the uterus. To prevent uterine overgrowth, progesterone slows this activity and redirects growth elsewhere. Your fertility doctor will augment your natural production of progesterone to avoid early miscarriage and help maintain a healthy level of progesterone during pregnancy. It stimulates bone growth, helping to protect from osteoporosis; helps maintain a healthy weight by burning body fat for energy; decreases craving for sweet and high-sugar foods, stabilising blood sugar levels. Is a diuretic, normalising body fluid and salt levels.

Different Forms of Progesterone
Vaginal suppositories
Widely used but are not FDA-approved. Wax-based, compounded by specialty pharmacists, used up to 2-3 times a day. Leakage can be messy.

Vaginal gel
This is the only once-daily FDA-approved progesterone for ART for up to 12 weeks of pregnancy This is also the only FDA-approved progesterone for a replacement for donor egg recipients and donor egg transfers. It's used once a day for progesterone supplementation. Some discharge reported during use.

Vaginal inserts: FDA-approved for progesterone supplementation but not for progesterone replacement. Effective in women under 35 years, used 2-3 times a day.

Injections: Widely used; the oldest, most established method for progesterone delivery, injected into the buttocks once a day. Requires a long, thick needle to penetrate layers of fat and skin. Injections may be painful. Difficult to administer by yourself.

Progesterone Side Effects During Pregnancy
In 1999, the FDA found that using synthetic progesterone may be associated with birth defects. Synthetic progesterone is primarily derived from the male hormone testosterone. Be very careful when undergoing progesterone treatments to make sure you're not using synthetic progesterone. Always consult a doctor when considering taking progesterone during pregnancy.

Common Side Effects When Using Progesterone
Drowsiness; fluid retention or bloating; hot flashes; depression; vaginal discharge; urinary problems; dizziness; abdominal pain or cramping; headaches; breast tenderness; joint pain.

Talking with your healthcare provider is important when deciding what supplementation is best for you. Progesterone supports implantation and pregnancy and is an important part of infertility treatment. Healthcare providers usually have a preference based on experience with other methods that can help you decide which supplementation is best for your infertility treatment.

Acupuncture to Aid Fertility

Acupuncture can increase fertility by reducing stress, increasing blood flow to the reproductive organs, and balancing the endocrine system, according to several studies and medical research. A recent study found that acupuncture, when used in conjunction with Western fertility treatments, increases conception rates by 26%.

Acupuncture works by stimulating nerve endings deep below the surface of the skin. By manipulating the needles in conjunction with gentle electrical stimulation (a practice known as electro puncture), your nerves are activated, helping your body release substances called endorphins. This can have positive effects on fertility, including relieving stress that may be weighing you down.

Acupressure points on the mid-section of the body - Ki 16: This is one of the most important acupuncture points for fertility. This reflexology point is located at one inch on both sides of the belly button. Stimulating this point is believed to improve general fertility health and boost the chances of conception in women.

According to the NHS, acupuncture is a treatment derived from traditional Chinese medicine where fine needles are inserted at certain points of the body for therapeutic or preventive purposes. This encourages the body to produce natural substances, such as pain-relieving endorphins and it's likely that these substances are responsible for the beneficial effects experienced by some from acupuncture.

How can Acupuncture Help Boost Fertility?

So, does acupuncture help boost your fertility naturally, when trying to conceive? According to a 2008 study by Edward Ernst, a Professor of Complementary Medicine, it was suggested that the acupuncture might help women to relax which would, in turn, improve pregnancy rates. It's important to note that this study was carried out on women undergoing IVF.

These theories suggest that acupuncture works by helping to release chemicals that send messages from the brain - called neurotransmitters - that affect reproductive hormones and organs; by stimulating blood flow to the uterus, thereby making embryo implantation more likely.

Natural Fertility

We will only briefly touch upon natural fertility here. As we said earlier, it is very important to us, but the purpose of this book is to sway gender.

It can be useful to try natural fertility treatments, like essential oils, to help get pregnant. Essential oils for conceiving can help regulate the body's natural rhythm and decrease stress to combat infertility. Using an essential oil diffuser can be especially effective in getting the mood just right, helping you relax, and ultimately promote fertility.

Topical application of these stress relief essential oils on the abdomen and lower back, and massage, are common ways to use essential oils to get pregnant. To help regulate menstruation, users can harness the natural benefits of lavender essential oil, clary sage essential oil, or rose essential oil to regulate periods and act as a natural medicine for ovulation. Lavender essential oil is thought to help relax muscles, improve circulation, and stimulate menstruation. The top essential oils for fertility are: Ylang Ylang, Clary Sage, Geranium, Fennel and Rose.

We would also like to touch upon Emotional Freedom Technique (EFT), better known as tapping, which is a technique that can be tied to ancient Chinese medicine. Tapping is the perfect tool when faced with infertility and can be used to control anxiety, for pain relief - both physical and emotional - for clearing limiting beliefs about your body, conception, pregnancy, childbirth, and parenthood and for installing new positive affirmations to make you feel empowered.

When we consciously slow down and check in with our bodies, our thoughts, and our feelings by using EFT, we open ourselves up to a wider perspective. EFT Tapping script for releasing negative beliefs while experiencing infertility: Say the following sentence out loud and rate how true it feels for you right now from 1 to 10, with 10 being it feels completely true: "I have faith in my body, and I trust that my spirit baby will arrive soon."

Pregnancy Testing and the Two Week Wait

We've all been there. Trying to conceive feels like a lifetime and consumes your every waking hour. It's one of the most precious yet nerve-wracking times in our life so it goes without saying we can't wait to see if our egg was fertilized, and the stork is preparing to descend carrying a new bundle of joy. Usually when ladies are trying to get pregnant many attempts are made – let's liken it to rabbits mating in the spring. A huge percentage of ladies don't track ovulation so they're not aware what DPO (days past ovulation) means, or how many DPO they are. They wait to see if their menstrual cycles begin, and if not, they'll take a pregnancy test.

The two primary methods are:

Testing for human pregnancy hormone (human chorionic gonadotropin - hCG) in blood or urine. Almost all pregnant women will have a positive urine pregnancy test one week after the first day of a missed menstrual period. What is very common in the gender sway world is early testing. You see it daily, ladies asking when people got a VVFL (very very faint line) or their BFP (big fat positive) and will start testing as early as 7dpo. Not only is this expensive (these tests aren't cheap). It also opens the doors for heartache if you experience a "chemical".

A chemical is also known as biochemical pregnancy or biochemical loss. It is the medical definition given to an early and spontaneous abortion or very early miscarriage. It's a normal pregnancy, in that conception happens after ovulation, the embryo implants, and a pregnancy test confirms the pregnancy. However, a miscarriage happens before the embryo or foetus can be seen in the uterus.

A chemical pregnancy is confirmed when an early pregnancy test reveals a positive result but later returns a negative result in a week or two. Sometimes the only real sign or symptom is a late period. Chemical pregnancies may account for 25–50 per cent of all miscarriages in cases when a person had no signs and didn't know they were pregnant. And those that don't test early who experience a chemical pregnancy never knew they were pregnant.

There's no right or wrong, we are all different, but we've seen and felt that heartache many times. To protect yourself emotionally it's always best to wait until the day your Aunt Flow is due to take that test.

Ready to Test?

You can carry out most pregnancy tests from the first day of a missed period. If you don't know when your next period is due, do the test at least 21 days after you last had unprotected sex. You can do a pregnancy test on a sample of urine collected at any time of the day. It doesn't have to be in the morning.

You can buy pregnancy testing kits from pharmacists and some supermarkets. They can give a quick result, and you can do the test in private. Most pregnancy tests come in a box that contains one or two long sticks. You pee on the stick and the result appears on the stick after a few minutes. All tests are slightly different, so always check the instructions.

A positive test result is almost certainly correct. However, a negative test result is less reliable. The result may not be reliable if you do not follow the instructions properly or take the test too early. Some medicines can also affect the results.

If you get a negative result and still think you're pregnant, wait a few days and try again. Speak to your GP to say if you get a negative result after a second test but your period has not arrived. We are here to support you emotionally through this, we have clients that also use BBT as the first indicator of pregnancy, followed by an implantation bleed. Implantation bleeding can be an early sign of pregnancy and just means your fertilised egg has implanted in the womb.

Things to Do in the Two Week Wait

Keep yourself busy, as focusing on whether you're pregnant or not will lead to anxiety and make the wait feel so much longer. We all do it, count down the days until we can test, and time stands still, like a child on Christmas Eve waiting for the morning to arrive and see if Santa has visited. It feels like an eternity. There's crafting, practising tarot readings or reading. Or organising things in the home, knowing that soon enough you will be reaching for the bucket, thanks to morning sickness and let's not mention the fatigue!

Think positively and do what you need to do whilst you still can. Why not add a little reiki too, which you can do easily at home through guided meditation? YouTube has some fantastic videos - get yourself comfortable and listen to the guide. One of our favourites is Divine Feminine Healing, Womb Blessings and Reiki for the Uterus.

We've also enrolled in an Astrology Diploma to further our knowledge, plus another course in Herbalism. Is there anything you've always wanted to do but just never got round to it? The perfect time to start is now. Make it an enjoyable time and look forward to pregnancy and gender joy.

Closing

Here we are, at the end of our natural sex selection book, but the beginning of your sway journey. We hope this book has opened you up to the intriguing world of natural sex selection, and that we've shown you the real science behind our method and how it all connects.

There will be days where you have doubts. And fear will get in your way. And that's ok! It happens to all of us. It did to us, too. But we did it! Our girls are our best friends. We kept our faith, and trust in the Zodiacs, and now you can too.

> *"Learn to trust the journey*
> *even when you don't understand it."*
> *- Mila Bron*

The evidence is overwhelming on the effects of the Moon and our emotional and physical body. We are confident in the benefits it has on fertility and gender selection. Facts speak for themselves, and we have plenty of those. Conceiving a child is a sacred bond and the ultimate act of commitment.

We are so happy to share this journey with you,

love Kelly and Claire x

www.cosmicswaymethod.com

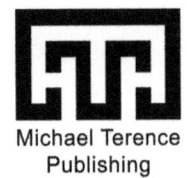

Michael Terence Publishing

www.mtp.agency

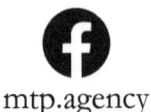

mtp.agency

@mtp_agency

www.ingramcontent.com/pod-product-compliance
Lightning Source LLC
LaVergne TN
LVHW051218070526
838200LV00064B/4962